AF832872

CARDIAC ARRHYTHMIAS - MECHANISMS, PATHOPHYSIOLOGY AND TREATMENT

Edited by **Wilbert S. Aronow**

Cardiac Arrhythmias - Mechanisms, Pathophysiology, and Treatment
http://dx.doi.org/10.5772/57008
Edited by Wilbert S. Aronow

Contributors

Bassel Suffian Al-Alao, B.C. Ramesh, Haralabos Parissis, Pascal Fallavollita, Ioana Mozos, Pavol Svorc, Ivana Bacova, Pavol Svorc, Jr., Monika Novakova, Alexander Marossy, Andrey Moskalenko, Wilbert S. Aronow

Published by InTech

Janeza Trdine 9, 51000 Rijeka, Croatia

Copyright © 2014 InTech

Individual chapters are under their authors' copyright and distributed under the Creative Commons Attribution 3.0 license, which allows users to download, copy and build upon published chapters provided that the authors and publisher are properly credited, which ensures maximum dissemination and a wider impact of the authors' work. Any republication, referencing or personal use of the individual chapters or any of their contents must explicitly identify the original source.

Permission for commercial use of the book as a whole, such as (but not limited to) reprint rights, republication, distribution, sales, translation, and reproduction in any and all forms of media, must always be obtained from InTech.

Notice

Statements and opinions expressed in the chapters are these of the individual contributors and not necessarily those of the editors or publisher. No responsibility is accepted for the accuracy of information contained in the published chapters. The publisher assumes no responsibility for any damage or injury to persons or property arising out of the use of any materials, instructions, methods or ideas contained in the book.

Publishing Process Manager Iva Lipovic

Technical Editor InTech DTP team

Cover InTech Design team

First published February, 2014

Printed in Croatia

Additional hard copies can be obtained from orders@intechopen.com

Cardiac Arrhythmias - Mechanisms, Pathophysiology, and Treatment, Edited by Wilbert S. Aronow

p. cm.

ISBN 978-953-51-1221-1

We are IntechOpen, the world's leading publisher of Open Access books

Built by scientists, for scientists

4,200+
Open access books available

116,000+
International authors and editors

125M+
Downloads

151
Countries delivered to

Our authors are among the
Top 1%
most cited scientists

12.2%
Contributors from top 500 universities

WEB OF SCIENCE™

Selection of our books indexed in the Book Citation Index in Web of Science™ Core Collection (BKCI)

Interested in publishing with us?
Contact book.department@intechopen.com

Numbers displayed above are based on latest data collected.
For more information visit www.intechopen.com

For EU product safety concerns:
IN TECH d.o.o., Prolaz Marije Krucifikse Kozulić 3, 51000 Rijeka, Croatia,
info@intechopen.com or visit our website at intechopen.com.

Meet the editor

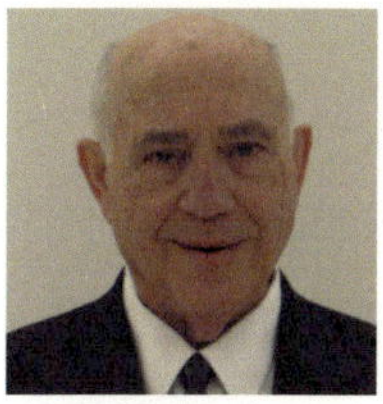

Wilbert S. Aronow, MD is Professor of Medicine at New York Medical College. Dr. Aronow has edited 12 books and is an author or coauthor of 1, 328 papers, 215 commentaries or Letters to the Editor, and 923 abstracts. He is currently a member of the Board of Directors of the American Society of Preventive Cardiology and a member of the American College of Chest Physicians Cardiovascular Disease, Hypertension, and Cardiovascular Surgery Network Steering Committee. He has been a member of 88 editorial boards of medical journals, co-editor of 2 journals, deputy editor of 1 journal, executive editor of 3 journals, an associate editor for 9 journals, and a guest editor for 7 other journals.

Contents

Preface

This book is a useful resource that every physician taking care of patients with cardiac arrhythmias should be familiar with. This book includes six chapters written by experts in their field.

Chapter 1 is a very comprehensive article on basic mechanisms of cardiac arrhythmias.

Chapter 2 discusses the chronobiological aspects of the impact of apnoic episodes on ventricular arrhythmias.

Chapter 3 focuses on the most recent developments in navigation, detection, and tracking during cardiac ablation interventions.

Chapter 4 discusses the epidemiology and pathophysiology of ventricular arrhythmias in several noncardiac diseases, the main methods used to assess arrhythmia risk, and their association with long-term outcomes. Dyslipidemia, diabetes mellitus, obesity, and liver, hematologic, neurologic, and psychiatric disorders are discussed.

Chapter 5 discusses the prevalence and prognosis of ventricular arrhythmias in patients with and without heart disease. Medical therapy including use of antiarrhythmic drugs and invasive intervention for complex ventricular arrhythmias are discussed. Studies on the effect of the automatic implantable cardioverter-defibrillator (AICD) on mortality in patients with ventricular tachyarrhythmias are discussed. Indications for implantation of an AICD for primary and for secondary prevention in patients with and without congestive heart failure are discussed.

Chapter 6 discusses surgical management of atrial fibrillation.

Financial and Competing Interests Disclosure

The author has no relevant affiliations or financial involvement with any organization or entity with a financial interest in or financial conflict with the subject matter or materials discussed in the manuscript. This includes employment, consultancies, honoraria, stock ownership or options, expert testimony, grants or patents received or pending, or royalties.

No writing assistance was utilized in the production of this manuscript.

Wilbert S. Aronow
Cardiology Division, Department of Medicine,
Westchester Medical Center/New York Medical College,
Valhalla, NY, USA

Chapter 1

Basic Mechanisms of Cardiac Arrhythmias[1]

Andrey Moskalenko

Additional information is available at the end of the chapter

http://dx.doi.org/10.5772/57557

1. Introduction

1.1. What should the activity of the heart and the action of the heart mean?

The term "*action of the heart*" was discussed in detail in my recent publication [1]. The terms "(any) cardiac activity" or "(any) activity of the heart" should be used only for designation any aimless functioning of the heart. On the other hand, "the action of the heart" or "the cardiac action" should be comprehended as the functioning of the heart that is directed to maintenance of physiological homeostasis, which is the target function in this case. Obviously, the action of the heart can be put into effect only due to a quantity of control loops and guidance loops[2], which all together organize one and indivisible cardiovascular system. Electrical phenomena, that accompany the functioning of the heart and can be recorded by electrocardiography, are nowise satisfying the target of the cardiovascular functioning, because they are but side effects of the *autowave function of the heart* [1, 2]. In English scientific and medical literature, the electrical phenomena to accompany the functioning of the heart are referred to as "the electrical *activity* of the heart" in a good accordance with the remarks above.

Any action of the heart that differs from its normal action ought to be ranked among *cardiac arrhythmias*. The normal action of the heart (the normal cardiac action) should be understood as the averaged round the human population cardiac behavior in comfort conditions. The cardiac arrhythmia arising in comfort conditions is undoubtedly considered to be pathologic. However, different kinds of cardiac arrhythmia arising in conditions distant from the comfort may be either *pathologic* cardiac behavior or normal *adaptive* response of the heart.

1This chapter is mainly based on our previous publication [2], which is revised and renewed for the aims of this book. The chapter contains some materials that have not been available previously to English-speaking readers.

2 Notice that the control is used to maintain a desired output of the system under control, while the guidance is intended for shifting the system from a state A to a state B.See more below.

INTECH
open science | open minds

© 2014 Moskalenko; licensee InTech. This is a paper distributed under the terms of the Creative Commons Attribution License (http://creativecommons.org/licenses/by/3.0), which permits unrestricted use, distribution, and reproduction in any medium, provided the original work is properly cited.

To make the proper diagnosis of arrhythmia type, one requires a deep understanding of the basic mechanisms of the cardiac action in being normal as well as in its various disorders.

1.2. Has the time come for alteration of the cardiologic paradigm?

Despite major scientific, medical and technological advances over the last few decades, a cure of cardiac arrhythmias remains elusive. As a very appropriate example of the problems of traditional cardiology, which is generally based on physiological approach, is the result of the CAST [3, 4], a multicenter, double-blind, randomized controlled trial, that has revealed a higher rate of death from arrhythmia of the patients treated with antiarrhythmic agents in comparison with the patients assigned to placebo. One of the well-known Russian cardiologists having analyzed a number of multicenter trials came to the conclusion [5] that treatment with antiarrhythmic drugs is prescribed nearly at random; he shared his impression with the following words[3]: "*Potentially any of the known antiarrhythmic drugs can 1) cause an antiarrhythmic effect, 2) not cause it, 3) be arrhythmogenic. And each of these cases happens unpredictably for a patient. Therefore, pharmacological tests are strongly required for selecting not only effective but, at least, harmless therapy for patients with malignant ventricular arrhythmias.*" Another author impressed by the result asserted that antiarrhythmic drugs have "*cost more American lives than the Vietnam War*" [6].

Another convincing example of the same is given to us by the recent discussion about the mechanisms of cardiac fibrillation [7]. The intensity of authors' disappointment is expressed by their writing that the nature of fibrillation remains "*still so puzzling after 160 years of inquiry*". A generally accepted definition of cardiac fibrillation is lacking.

Hence, it remains to add that the history of science gives a lot of resembling examples convincing us that the actual state of affairs suggests a self-evident necessity of drastic alteration of the scientific paradigm that forms the basis of modern cardiology.

1.3. The physiological description of the heart

The discovery of "animal electricity" must undoubtedly be recognized as a very important step in understanding the causes and mechanisms of cardiac disorders. Furthermore, this discovery quickly led to the development of a new language, the *physiological language*, which appeared to be very convenient for a generalized description of such properties of living matter that had been believed to be absolutely different before.

Indeed, what common features between functions of the brain and of the muscles can be found out by somebody without special knowledge? What common, it would seem, can be between muscular power and the power of thought? However, the discovery of the "animal electricity" allowed registering a certain process that can be observed both in nervous and in muscle

3 In the original: «потенциально любой из известных антиаритмических препаратов может: а) обеспечить антиаритмический эффект; б) не обеспечить его; в) проявить аритмогенное действие. И все это индивидуально непредсказуемо. Поэтому для больных со злокачественными желудочковыми аритмиями выбор не только эффективной, но и безопасной терапии требует проведения фармакологических проб» [Голицын С.П. Грани пользы и риска при лечении желудочковых нарушений ритма сердца. Международный журнал медицинской практики 2000;(10) 56–64].

tissues; the process was given the name "excitation". Since then the nervous and muscle tissues have been referred to as "excitable tissues". Further development of ideas about excitable tissues made scientists draw some extremely important generalizations of all those experimental data which were collected by the end of the 19th century. It was as long ago as 1900 [8] that T.W. Engelmann, K.F. Wenckebach and H.P. Bowditch postulated the basic properties of the myocardium, namely: 1) automaticity, 2) refractory period, 3) all-or-nothing response, 4) staircase phenomenon. It is the concept of "animal electricity" that has formed the basis for all the subsequent physiological investigations.

Here we will not dwell on the peculiarities of the physiological language used for description of biological objects, as these are written in many textbooks of physiology quite a lot and in detail (for example, see [8–10]). It should only be emphasized that, after replacing the old notion of a special "living substance", the physiological language has entirely dominated among biologists and medical professionals for the whole 20th century.

However, the discussion between modern investigators of the heart reveals faultiness of the cardiologic paradigm, which is constructed owing to the epoch-making discoveries made by the greatest physiologists of the 19th and 20th centuries. The faultiness appears to be caused by our rather simple comprehension how biological systems work, which arose from the historic specificity of scientific knowledge evolution. During 17–19th centuries the science development is known to be mainly grounded on the notions of determinism, with great advantage in applied mechanics to constitute their historical basis. It resulted in permeating the conception, which is referred to as *mechanistic approach*[4] now, into many fields of science. Nor has medicine escaped the common lot, since all modern physiology is per se a manifestation of the mechanistic approach in biology. In accordance with scientific tradition, the phenomena observed in physiology are explained, in the frames of the mechanistic approach, as a result of different simple mechanical movements. The movement of ions through membrane of a biological cell in order to explain the action potential is a good example of the approach. Prevalent endeavors of modern cardiologists to treat cardiac disorders by adjusting membrane channels using one or another drug is another such example.

More and more researchers [11–15] are coming to an increasingly profound understanding that there is a need for an alternative or modified paradigm, in order to consider the multi-systemic nature of the body's function and its environmental interface if new and more effective therapies are to be developed. Recognizing a problem is the first step to its solution...

1.4. Cardiophysics

Over the past few decades, it have been accumulated quite a large number of experimental observations and theoretical results which are poorly fit within the constraints set by the physiological language. These new discoveries were called attention to, which has resulted in both drawing new generalizations of the collected scientific knowledge and developing a new

4 To distinguish the "mechanistic approach" and "insight into mechanisms" is extremely important. In the terms of mathematical physics, the mechanistic approach is based on linear description of nature, with the principle of superposition being correct in the frames of this approach; however, non-linear mechanisms are shown to underlie a huge number of natural phenomena (for example, see [16, 17]), and, hence, insight into such non-linear mechanisms is also very desired.

language, the *biophysical* one. For example, while the physiological approach fails to take chaotic dynamics into account, the biophysical way of living system description, mainly based on the theory of dynamical system, has equipped scientists with reliable quantitative methods of studying enorganic phenomena of deterministic chaos. Modern scientific disciplines lead to the conclusion that often adequate comprehension of a complex system requires analyzing not the observed values, but some of its integral characteristics, which can be mathematically obtained as a combination of a number of the observed. Chaotic attractor is a good illustration of how important ideas of modern physics are for cardiology [16–18]. Whether any sort of chaotic attractors correspond to the normal cardiac activity, remains still a very good question. Other crucial phenomena that must certainly be taken into account when treatment for a cardiologic patient is provided are caused by so-called "bifurcation memory", which has attracted special attention of investigators since recently [19–21]. Recent evidence suggests that similar phenomena can be found in the heart [1, 2]. The results of investigating the bifurcation memory in a cardiac model are presented and discussed below.

The following three other examples are intended to illustrate how the use of new biophysical laws has led to a substantially deeper understanding of well-known phenomena, not achievable within the frames of physiology.

Experimental results from studies in electro- and magnetocardiology gave rise to the modern biophysical conception of "*equivalent bioelectric generator*" [22], which is strongly based on classical electrodynamics. The first example is to demonstrate how the conception of "equivalent bioelectric generator" was useful for investigation of the QT dispersion problem. QT dispersion (QTD) is simply defined as the difference between the longest (QTmax) and the shortest (QTmin) QT intervals within a 12-lead ECG; since its description in 1990, it has been considered as "undergoing vigorous assessment" for the purpose of early identifying subjects at high risk of sudden cardiac death, because it was supposed that "the interlead QT interval differences within a 12-lead ECG might reflect regional differences in myocardial refractoriness, and that this might predict cardiac dysrhythmias" [23]. Common sense based on the physiological concept seemed to point quite convincingly to the prognostic significance of the phenomenon of QTD, because it is expected that electrophysiological instability of activation and recovery of the myocardium must necessarily be reflected on the surface of the torso in a form of instability of ECG-patterns of the repolarization part of the cardiac cycle. In spite of that, the accurate, from the standpoint of biophysics, study of possible mechanisms of QTD, after problems of the QT-interval genesis were considered in terms of biophysical models of the cardiac electric activity, has led to the conclusion that the duration of the QT-interval (tQT) are the same in each electrocardiographic leads, and the "QT dispersion" phenomenon stems mainly from mistakes in detecting the T-wave end [24, 25]. Electrical activity of the ventricular myocardium in such models is determined only by the equivalent cardiac dipole, which the spatial vector loops QRS and T correspond to. Although the normal work of the heart can be successfully described by a dipole, multipole components are given rise to when cardiac disorders occur. It can be stated therefore that the phenomenon of QTD reflects the contribution of the multipole components in a total picture of the electrical activity of the heart. Let us denote duration of QT in different leads as tQT(l), where l belongs to a set of leads L. The theoretical consideration within the dipole hypothesis has showed [24] that the QT-duration in different leads, tQT(l), must be exactly equal to each other with the exception, perhaps, of some *very special cases* as well as that, at a low noise level and, consequently, the low threshold of identification the end of the T-wave, it is difficult to expect a large spread of the values tQT(l) measured from leads to leads in a case of vector loops with a *finite radius of curvature*. The differences in tQT(l) observed in practice can be explained only by algorithms used for detecting the T-wave end or the ECG isoline, by choice of the thresholds of identification in relation to the accepted rules of coding the presence of the ECG-waves, or by the actual values of the signal / noise ratio, as well as by measurement errors. Nevertheless, the authors identified a number of factors [25] that can even within the dipole hypothesis result in increasing dispersion of QT-duration both in a sequence of cardiocycles from the same leads and in a set of records of the same cardiac cycle simultaneously registered in the different leads. Two most significant factors are following:

1. There is no clear correspondence between the positions of electrical and anatomical axes of the heart due to physiologically normal variations in topography of His-Purkinje system.

2. QT-dispersion also depends on the random rotations of the ventricles relative to the measuring electrodes, for example, during rotation of the heart relative to its anatomical axes.

Hence, the investigation [24, 25] has shown that it is impossible at present to reject the hypothesis of random nature of the QTD changes, since all of these factors that generate QTD changes should be considered as random variables. Regardless of the biophysical result, it is still believed, however, that "increased QT dispersion is associated with increased risk of cardiovascular death" [26].

The second example deals with defibrillation. Cardiologists are known to have been working on the problem of defibrillation for several decades, but desired level of success has not yet been achieved, and the fundamental mechanisms that underlie defibrillation still remain a mystery [27]. At present there is no generally accepted point of view on the mechanisms of postshock arrhythmia induction resulting from unsuccessful defibrillation. A number of factors were assumed among the possible causes of an unsuccessful defibrillation; for example: 1) residual fibrillation activity in areas of weak voltage gradient, 2) new autowave vortices generated by a shock, 3) focal ectopic activity in areas of myocardium traumatized the action of electric current that a defibrillator produces. Suggested in the last years, the new Theory of Virtual Electrodes [28, 29] helps to understand failures of the defibrillation protocols presently in use. One of the most important practical conclusions of the theory is the recommendation to use a biphasic defibrillation stimulus, which can significantly increase the effectiveness of defibrillation. It should be noted that the emergence of new look at defibrillation and the subsequent development of the theory of virtual electrodes became possible only by using one of the fresher biophysical models of such intricate active medium as the myocardium, which is referred to "bidomain model". In addition, several researches [30, 31], which also are carried out in the frames of cardiophysical approach, are aimed at developing new techniques of defibrillation based on suppression of cardiac turbulent dynamics by weak local excitations.

Returning to the results of CAST and other similar investigation, we ought to remind that these results were evident directly from the very early theoretical works of those scientists who can undoubtedly be mentioned among the founders of a new branch of science, cardiophysics. First of all, I mean here the studies by Arthur Winfree [32], who has revealed the principal autowave regimes of the simplest active medium and their dependence on the basic integral parameters of the medium, as well as by Valentin Krinsky and Iury Kokoz [33], who have shown that every active medium should demonstrate the same set of principal autowave regimes, because the corresponding systems of partial differential equation can always be reduced to the simplest one. Taken together these results lead to the obvious conclusion that any manipulation with the membrane ion channels of cardiomyocytes directed to the suppression of ventricular tachycardia by forcing autowave vortices to perform uniform circular motion (which corresponds to monomorphic tachycardia) always results in to the displacement of myocardial state very far from normal, which must inevitably increase patient mortality. Note that the hypothesis about the displacement of myocardial state was confirmed later in an experimental work with lidocaine [34], in good accordance with Winfree's prediction. Another biophysical study [35] demonstrated one more reason why medicines that exhibit strongly pronounced antiarrhythmic properties when affecting single cardiomyocyte increase in 2-3 times the frequency of sudden arrhythmic death in comparison to untreated patients. At first glance, it does seem paradoxical that the same drug has antiarrhythmic effect on isolated cells and pro-arrhythmic effect on the multicellular system (the whole heart). In the computational imitating experiments, the author managed nevertheless to discover that sodium channel blockers can greatly increase the so-called vulnerable period in myocardium, which occurs because of a decrease of velocity of the excitation wave, and also because of reduction of excitability gradient. The next remark deals with ECG diagnostics. Notwithstanding the properties of myocardium are known to affect ECG, the investigation of the dependence of several ECG characteristics on the threshold of excitation, which was carried out by means of mathematical modeling monomorphic arrhythmias in a homogeneous two-dimensional excitable medium, revealed [36] that these arrhythmias appear under both decreased and increased values of the excitation threshold. Hence, this result leads also to the conclusion that medical treatments are prescribed nearly at random when a cardiologist make his or her decision only on the base of ECG analysis without knowing about real changes of the excitation threshold. Generalizing these three biophysical conclusions about medical treatment of tachycardia, should we be surprised that the success of such treatment can hardly be called acceptable?

In addition to remarkable progress in biophysics, another important conceptual breakthrough of science was performed in the field that now is referred to as *nonequilibrium thermodynamics*, *"physics of becoming"* [37] or *synergetics* [38], which "represents a remarkable confluence of many strands of thought, and has become a paradigm in modern culture" [39]. Biological systems are complex and nonlinear, and, therefore, demonstrate complex and nonlinear behavior, which may be chaotic, in many cases; the heart appears to be the same [14, 17, 18, 28, 30, 31].

All these examples should be recognized as proofs of birth of a new science. Thus, we ought to conclude that the 21st century seems to yield a new discipline, which is referred to as *cardiovascular physics*[5] or *cardiophysics* (since it combines cardiology with novel achievements of physics). Cardiophysics is an interdisciplinary science that stands at the junction of cardiology and biophysics, with researchers using the methods of, and theories from, physics to study cardiovascular system at different levels of its organization, from the molecular scale to whole organisms. Being formed historically as part of systems biology, cardiophysics is designed to reveal connections between the physical mechanisms, underlying the organization of the cardiovascular system, and biological features of its functioning.

2. Basic biophysical mechanisms of maintaining the action of the heart

2.1. Historical remarks

About fifty year ago, physicists and mathematicians managed to perceive that the processes that take place in a "purely physical" systems (e.g., lasers, or even in boiling water) are similar in some of their properties to the processes observed in the physiology of excitable biological tissues. The understanding came gradually that phenomena such as irritability, conductivity, all-or-nothing response, refractory period etc. are inherent not only exclusively in biological objects, but also typical for non-living nature. It is important to comprehend that the speech here is not about some analogies, but exactly about a new scientific generalization of the accumulated scientific knowledge, and that the generalization made by researchers in respect of particular types of behavior of living and some non-living systems is based on the certain entirely real properties of such systems. This generalization led to the development of a new language, biophysical one, which are more universal and more powerful. The new language has reproduced the description of all that was already described earlier in the physiology, but it also allows in unified terms to represent a wide range of experimental data, the description of which the physiological language performed poorly. The new expanded description of the cardiac action is offered in this chapter further.

Undoubtedly, the term *"autowave"*, which refers to a large number of different biological objects, plays one of the most important roles in the new biophysical language.

The first who studied actively the self-oscillations was Academician A.A. Andronov, and the term *"auto-oscillations"* in Russian terminology was introduced by him in 1928. The term *"autowaves"* was proposed in the second half of the 20th century, probably, on the analogy of the previously used "auto-oscillations". The classical axiomatic model of autowaves in myocardium was published in 1946 by Norbert Wiener and Arturo Rosenblueth [40]. During 1970-80, major efforts to study autowaves were concentrated in the Institute of Biological Physics of the USSR Academy of Sciences. A huge role in the study of autowave models of cardiac tissue belongs to D. Noble and members of his team from the University of Oxford [12, 13]. There are a lot of other researchers over the world who contributed to development of the

5 For example, there are already the Group of Nonlinear Dynamics & Cardiovascular Physics of the 1st Faculty of Mathematics and Natural Sciences in the Institute of Physics of Humboldt University of Berlin (German) and the Cardiovascular Biophysics Laboratory in Washington University (USA).

theory of the autowave processes, i.e. the processes in the *active media*. Since then, as the peculiar properties of the active media has been understood, the autowave processes attract attention of mathematicians, physicists and biologists, and it turned out, that the experience that had been gained by physiologists before gave a very useful basis for constructing the new biophysical language for describing phenomena observed in the active media of different nature.

2.2. Mathematical aspects

According to [41], the term "*autowaves*" is used for designation of a self-sustaining nonlinear undulatory process in a non-equilibrium (active) medium, the process remaining unchanged for sufficiently small changes in both the initial and boundary conditions and described by the system of parabolic partial differential equations with a nonlinear free member, which in its general form can be written as follows: $\vec{u}_t = \vec{f}(\vec{u}) + D\Delta\vec{u}$, where $\vec{u}$ is a vector of state variables, $\vec{u}_t$ is the time derivative of the $\vec{u}$, $\vec{f}(\vec{u})$ is a vector of free members (i.e., of nonlinear functions), D is a diagonal matrix of the coefficients that describe diffusion of each component, and Δ is the Laplace operator. Thus, the mathematical apparatus that are often used for describing autowave processes are the equations of the diffusion type with an active nonlinearity (i.e. *reaction–diffusion systems*).

It is impossible here to delve into the details of the mathematical description of autowave processes, but there are an abundance of literature on this topic (for example, see [32, 33, 40–47]). Therefore only those aspects which are the most important for understanding the nature of cardiac arrhythmias will be touched on here. To apprehend distinctly the signification of the term "autowaves", several things should be noted.

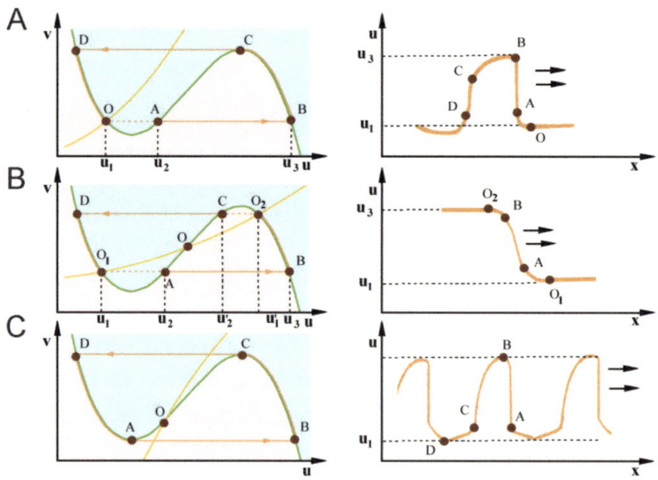

Figure 1. Phase portraits (left column) and the corresponding behavior (right column) of a single element of the active medium: row **A** — excitable, row **B** — bistable, row **C** — self-oscillating element types. Rose area corresponds to $f_1(u, v)>0$, and blue color highlights the area, where $f_1(u, v)<0$. See description in the text.

First of all, a general property of such systems, regardless of whether they are of animate or of inanimate nature, is that they consist of external energy sources distributed in the space; and such special systems were called *"active media"*. From the thermodynamic point of view, these are open systems far from thermodynamic equilibrium [41]. It is the quality that compels the behavior of the active media to differ fundamentally from that of systems which have been familiar to physicists of the 19th and 20th centuries. Even the waves in active media propagate according to essentially different laws than the well-known acoustic or electromagnetic waves do. Unlike linear waves — such as sound waves, electromagnetic waves and other, which are inherent in conservative systems and mathematically described by linear second order hyperbolic equations (wave equations), — dynamics of an autowave in terms of differential equations can be described by *parabolic equation with nonlinear free member of a special form* (the equation is presented at a few lines above).

It was shown in 1973 [33] that every system of mathematical differential equations describing the process of excitation of biological tissues can be simplified with use of some standard mathematical procedures to only two equations that describe, with an acceptable accuracy, the real object for which the "exact" original system of many equations was composed. It proved that such systems are a very important kind of active media, which has been called *"active media with recovery"* (note, that nerve impulse, which serves typical example of autowaves in the active medium with recovery, was studied as far back as 1850 by Hermann von Helmholtz). Thus, the following system of two equations is recognized to be the base model of the active medium with recovery [41]:

$$\varepsilon \cdot u_t = f_1(u,v) + D_1 \Delta u \tag{1}$$

$$v_t = f_2(u,v) + D_2 \Delta v \tag{2}$$

where $\varepsilon << 1. D_2 = 0$ for excitable biological membranes, whereas both the diffusion coefficient, D_1 and D_2, are different from zero for chemical systems. For biological membranes, the meaning of the variables of state is as follows: u corresponds to the membrane potential, and v is the conductivity of the slow component of the membrane current. Although the exact description of a specific sort of active medium can take much more equations (for example, the modern model of the human myocardium consists of more than twenty equations), the most important basic properties of autowave processes are well described already within this basic model of active media.

The next essential moment is that the active media are characterized not only by the connections between the adjacent points of the medium (i.e. by flows of substances and / or energy, such as heat conduction or diffusion, which is described by $D\Delta\vec{u}$ in the system of equations).The concrete form of the free member $\vec{f}(\vec{u})$ is of exceptional importance, because all wave processes are generated by the nonlinear dynamics of the point system $\vec{u}_t = \vec{f}(\vec{u})$, which always must be self-oscillating or potentially self-oscillating. In the base model of the active medium with recovery, the complicated nonlinear behavior of a single element is described by the free member, i.e. as the function $f_1(u, v)$, which usually has **N**-shaped form (Figure 1). Three simplest types of such elements can be distinguished [17, 42, 43]; one can also say that a single element has three essentially different regimes of its behavior, because it is possible to force the element change its type. These are: *self-excited* (or *self-oscillating*), *excitable* (or *waiting*) and *trigger* (or *bistable*) regimes. Accordingly, there are three types of homogeneous active media composed of these elements.

The *excitable* element (row **A** of Figure 1) has only one stable steady state (the point **O**, which is the intersection of the two null isoclines; a quiescent state of the excitable element corresponds with this point). External impact over a threshold level (i.e., greater than the length of the segment **OA**), can bring the excitable element out from its steady state and force it accomplish a certain evolution (in the phase portrait shown by the orange line) before returning to its quiescent state. An excited element may affect the adjacent elements moving them out from their quiescent state. As a result, an autowave of excitation spreads through the medium. Excitable media like the working myocardium consist of such excitable elements. Hence, it becomes obvious the fallacy of popular opinion that "all cardiac cells have spontaneous firing capacity, but only at a very slow heart rate", the assertion which can be often met in books and papers.

The *bistable* element (row **B** of Figure 1) has two steady states at the points $\mathbf{O_1}$ and $\mathbf{O_2}$, each of which can be whether stable or unstable, while the point O in this case is always unstable. Transitions between the two stationary states occur when an external impact exceeds a certain threshold level (the same way as it does in the excitable element). In such media there can be the *trigger wave* propagation, which switches the media from one steady state to the other. A classic case of such a switching autowave (and, perhaps, the simplest autowave phenomena) is falling dominoes. Another simple example of the bistable medium is burning paper: the switching wave propagates on it in the form of a flame, switching paper from the normal state to its ashes.

The *self-oscillating* element (row **C** of Figure 1) has no stable steady states (the point O in this case is always unstable) and therefore it permanently performs oscillations of certain fixed form, amplitude and frequency. An example of a self-oscillating medium is the sinus node of the heart, in which excitation impulses arise spontaneously. External influence can disturb these oscillations, but, after some relaxation time, all their characteristics, except for the phase, revert to the stable values, although the phase can be changed, resulting in the phase waves spread in the self-excited medium. Such phase waves can be observed in electro-garlands or in certain chemical media.

So it can be clearly seen on the phase portrait of the basic system of equations describing active medium of different types (see Figure 1) that a significant difference between these three types of behavior of an active medium is caused by the quantity and the position of its singular points. The shapes of autowaves observed in reality can be, however, very similar to each other, and therefore it can be difficult to assess correctly the type of element only by the form of its excitation impulse.

http://dx.doi.org/10.5772/57557

It is reasonable that a good number of examples of combined active media, which are composed of different types of elements, can be found everywhere. The heart is just one example of a highly organized combined active medium.

2.3. Pacemakers

The region of a combined active medium which consists of self-oscillatory elements is called the *pacemaker*. This region emits autowaves with a certain stable period. An example of a biological pacemaker in the heart of the human is the sinus node, which is constituted of a group of cells functioning in the self-oscillating mode.

In thin enough layers of the active medium, the pacemaker creates a picture in the form of ring waves diverging from a center (Figure 2). Period of pacemaker oscillations is determined by its intrinsic properties and can be arbitrary, but not less than the absolute refractory period, because a new action potential cannot arise during the absolute refractory period (see below).

If there are a number of self-oscillating elements with different periods in the medium, every element with low-frequency activity is suppressed by the element with the highest frequency [41]. For a long time physiologists have known about the hierarchy of pacemakers in the heart, and the same result was obtained mathematically in the second half of twentieth century. Pacemakers in the heart are the sinoatrial (SA) node, the atrioventricular (AV) node and the bundle of His and Purkinje fibers. The sinoatrial node normally initiates action potentials, simply because it generates impulses slightly faster than the other areas with self-oscillating activity. The remaining pacemakers normally are in a depressed state, which is reflected by physiological language as "latent pacemaker capability." If the SA node is suddenly "out of order", the fastest of the "spare" pacemakers (i.e., the AV node) enters into work, and, as a result, the heart continues its action nearly in normal regime. This duplication of parts of the system is aimed, evidently, to improve its reliability.

However, recent studies [49, 50] have shown that the rhythmic activity of the self-oscillating elements in the group which form the body of the pacemaker is synchronized by more complex laws, and the ascertained earlier variant of synchronization from the element with the highest frequency of the oscillations is only a special case. The problem of the control of cardiac rhythm has been considered in terms of the general theory of the synchronization of relaxation systems, and, as result, the main pathways of the control of cardiac rhythm have been revealed: (1) control with regard for the features of synchronization of relaxation systems during the formation of the unified heart rhythm due to the acceleration of the slow diastole depolarization phase; (2) control by gradual integral increase in the duration of the slow diastole depolarization phase; (3) subsequent synchronization of the rhythm as a delay of the slow diastole depolarization phase.

2.4. Traveling autowaves

The concept "*traveling autowave*" (or "*autowave of excitation*", or "*propagating autowave*") should be considered as generalization made in the new biophysical language of the concept "excitation wave", which is understood in the frames of physiology as an electrical wave that

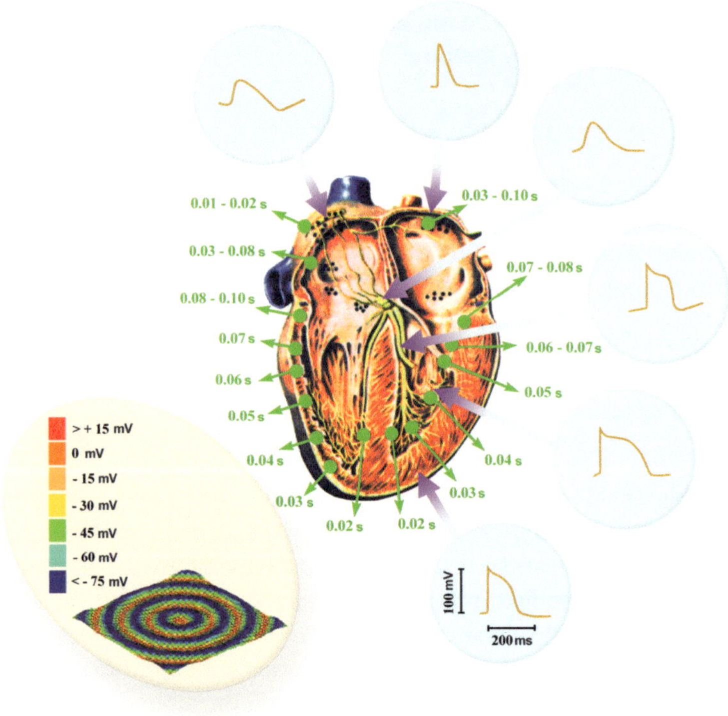

Figure 2. Spatiotemporal organization of the normal cardiac action. Green inscriptions and arrows indicate the time of arrival of the excitation wave in the corresponding region of the heart (using the data published in [48]). Blue incuts show the shape of the traveling wave ("action potential") in different areas of the heart caused by the difference in properties of the elements of the excitable medium that forms the heart tissue. Beige incut demonstrates the normal propagation of the traveling-wave of excitation from the pacemaker area in the center (from the sinus node) towards the edges (through the working myocardium) in a simple simulation model.

propagates along a muscle fiber just before its contraction. Autowaves of excitation are perhaps the most common in nature autowave phenomena, they occur in a variety of physical, chemical and biological objects. According to the earliest investigations [40–42], "traveling autowave" was a designation of the wave processes that have stable ("self-sustaining") parameters, such as speed, amplitude, and pulse shape, independently of initial conditions. It was believed also that "if two autowaves propagate toward each other, they do not pass through each other, like linear waves and solitons do it, but they annihilate in a collision" [41]. Autowaves was believed to be not able to interfere or to reflect from obstacles. These properties were considered as a significant difference of autowaves from the usual electromagnetic or sound waves.

Analysis of the systems of mathematical equations that describe the active medium has given not only a quite good explanation of the phenomena known from physiology, but also has led to the discovery of many new interesting properties of the active media, even in the earliest works. For example, the dependence of the traveling autowave velocity on the curvature of its front was obtained as a result of this analysis: the velocity decreases with increasing curvature, and there is a *critical value of the curvature*, above which the excitation wave propagation becomes impossible. For example, see [41, 47, 51–53]. The *critical curvature* leads, in particular, to the fact that the excitation autowaves can not pass through an aperture of sufficiently small size in a non-excitable obstacle (e.g., in the postinfarction scar). Other properties of traveling autowaves associated with critical curvature underlie different mechanisms of reentrant tachycardias, which will be considered in more details below.

Another interesting property of active media, which was found out in the earliest works, is that, for periodic autowaves, their velocity decreases with increasing frequency, and explicit expressions for calculating its value were derived. In such a way, it has been shown mathematically that the stationary propagation of autowaves is possible only as long as the wave period T is more than a certain value T_{min}, and that there is a certain mathematical dependence of the wave velocity on the medium properties [54, 55]. When $T < T_{min}$, the propagation occurs in some peculiar manner: though the excitation waves propagate without attenuation, not all of them propagate, but only, for example, every third or fourth wave, depending on T, which is known in cardiology as *Wenckebach periodicity*.

The existence of T_{min} is caused by the fact that the excitation autowave can not propagate until the recovery processes, which are described with the slow variable of the base model, has finished. This property of active media is called refractoriness, and the typical recovery time is called the refractory period.[6] *Refractoriness* is the fundamental property of any object of autowave nature (especially excitable medium) not to respond on stimuli, if the object stays in the specific refractory state. In common sense, *refractory period* is the characteristic recovery time, i.e. the period of time that is associated with the motion of the image point on the left branch of the isoclinic curve $u_t = 0$ (i.e. the segment DO; see row **A** of Figure 1). The *relative refractory period* is understood as the immediately following interval during which initiation of the next action potential is inhibited but not impossible. In the *state of relative refractoriness*, propagation of the next autowave is possible also before the full recovery of the media, but with slightly less velocity depending on the time elapsed since the passage of the previous wave. For periodic pulse, this results in *dispersion*, which is dependence of the autowave velocity on their frequency [44, 56]. If the time interval after the passage of the previous wave is too short, then propagation of the subsequent wave is impossible, so that, for every excitable medium, there is a certain minimal interval between a couple of successive waves, the absolute refractory period. The absolute refractory period is the interval during which the next action potential absolutely cannot be initiated, no matter how large a stimulus is applied. But, even in a fully recovered excitable medium, velocity of the excitation autowaves can not exceed a certain value, which is the maximum value for the medium and which is equal to the velocity of the traveling autowave of zero curvature (i.e. with the flat front, the *flat autowave*). The mathematical details can be found in the suggested literature.

---

6 Let us recall that the existence of the refractory period in the cardiac muscle has been ascertained as long as 1876 by EJ Marey, who was an extremely gifted French researcher in the physiology of the heart. It was he, who also introduced this term as well as who noted that the refractory period of the cardiac muscle lasts conspicuously longer than in skeletal muscle or nerve. In 1906, A.J. Carlson was the first who used the terms "absolute refractory period" and "relative refractory period"[8].

A lot of active media are characterized by the pronounced *relaxantness*, i.e. the time interval of refractoriness is noticeably longer than the time interval of excitation. In the basic model of the active medium with recovery, relaxantness is determined by a small parameter ε [41]. For cardiac tissue, the refractory period exceeds the excitation time approximately 300 times. This leads to the fact that the excitation wave in the heart has a sharp front edge, but has no pronounced trailing edge. The presence of prolonged refractoriness allows to explain, for example, the *annihilation* of the excitation waves when they collide. Because of long refractory tail, where the excitation is not possible, two waves can not pass through each other and die.

However, more recent studies [57–59] have shown that autowaves can exhibit more complicated behavior, and the properties described in the early classical works are observed only in a number of special cases. For example, it was found out that annihilation does not always occur in a collision of autowaves, but under certain conditions autowaves can pass through each other like solitons. Diffraction, reflection and splitting are also possible to observe for autowaves under certain conditions. It was shown that autowave shape and velocity may vary during its spontaneous evolution caused by the bifurcation memory [20, 21]. It was declared [20]:"The general theory of active media remains to be formulated, and practically each in-depth study reveals new types of their dynamics and self-organization. There is no reason to think that these types are unique; on the contrary, the available experience indicates that, once described, a new dynamic regime or bifurcation is thereafter found in other systems, even those that have been investigated for a long time". So it can be expected that further deepening of our knowledge of the properties of autowaves will also help us to understand the failure in the treatment of cardiac arrhythmias.

2.5. Spatiotemporal organization of the normal cardiac action

The main goal of the normal cardiac action is the pumping function of the heart. It is the ordered propagation of the excitation autowave in the myocardium that maintains efficient contraction of the heart, thereby allowing blood to be pumped throughout the body. For the pumping function of the heart to be maintained effective, appropriate *spatiotemporal organization* (STO) of the excitation process is extremely important. The appropriate STO is caused by the very structure of the heart, i.e. by the special spatial arrangement of various autowave elements (cardiomyocytes) with significantly different behavior (which, as mentioned above, is described with use of the nonlinear free member $\vec{f}(\vec{u})$ in the base model of the active medium with recovery). Due to the special spatial structure of the heart as a whole organ, well-known from courses of anatomy and physiology, the only mode of traveling waves initiated from the sinoatrial node occurs in the normal heart during the normal cardiac activity (Figure 2).

It is disorders of the spatiotemporal organization of the process of myocardial excitation and contraction that should be understood as a generalized mechanism of cardiac arrhythmias, which usually manifests with various electrical indications used by doctor to set the correct diagnosis. Note that these ideas are being developed in the concept of the autowave function of the heart [1], which has not yet received a rigorous mathematical formulation.

The simplest examples of disorders of the appropriate STO are various conduction block. The mechanism of partial conduction block has been described above from the biophysical

http://dx.doi.org/10.5772/57557

standpoint. The so called electrical conduction system of the heart should be considered only as an illusive perception of the real complicated active media that builds the body of the heart. The illusion is caused by sincere desire to describe the heart strictly within the frames of the mechanistic approach, which requires that some specific electric wires were searched for. However, there are not any electric wires in the cardiac tissue, which rather presents the network of active elements of different types. Each of these elements can be forced change its type by influence of humoral, nervous or metabolic factors. The target function of the inherent circulatory regulation consists in maintaining the appropriate STO independently from uncontrolled influence of humoral, nervous or metabolic factors. In those cases where the regulation is untenable, pathological states develop leading to disease. For example, additional sources of autowaves, arising from pathological changes of certain areas of the myocardium, can result in severe cardiac arrhythmias.

It is extremely important to understand that the function $\vec{f}(\vec{u})$ may be changed in the same way at various combinations of values of the individual parameters of the cardiomyocyte, but even utterly different combinations of individual parameters may result in the same clinical manifestations of cardiac disorders inasmuch as they are determined by the state of the function $\vec{f}(\vec{u})$ rather than by any of the individual parameters of the myocardium. It is not sodium, potassium, calcium, etc. conductivity of membrane ion channels in cardiomyocytes (as it is usual for physiologists to think) causes the normal cardiac action, but exactly that of their combinations which is optimal for the given conditions of functioning of the organism. It is likely that causes of the cases of unsuccessful pharmacological treatment of cardiac arrhythmias, which were revealed, particularly, in CAST, hide themselves somewhere here.

Hence, cardiac arrhythmia should be considered in a more general way: they occur either as a consequence of disorders of STO, or as a consequence of disorders in inherent circulatory regulation, but not as isolated disorders of the cardiac electrical activity.

3. Basic biophysical mechanisms of cardiac arrhythmias

Since autowave processes were pointed in the role of sources of cardiac arrhythmias, the number of known types of sources of cardiac arrhythmias has increased significantly. This increase is associated not only with discovery of a number of new mechanisms of arrhythmias, but also with distinction of the mechanisms that were equated with each other before. So for *reentry*, a mechanism of arrhythmias known since the 19th century, it is accepted to distinguish now at least five types: (1) running around a ring, (2) spiral wave, (3) autowave reverberator, (4) multiple reverberators, and (5) fibrillation as chaotic behavior of autowave reverberators. In accordance with the classification of principal mechanisms of cardiac arrhythmias that was suggested in [60], the running around a ring as well as the spiral wave should be reckoned among *anatomic reentry*, while the others belong to *functional reentry*.

Altered automaticity, which is the second classical mechanism of arrhythmogenesis, can be divided into (1) *altered normal* automaticity, (2) *abnormal* (or induced) automaticity, and (3) *triggered activity*. Regarding *increased automaticity*[7], several new types of automatic nature were also discovered, in addition to the pacemaker activity. These are: (1) induced automaticity, (2) *leading center*, (3) triggered activity by the mechanism of *early afterdepolarization*, and (4) triggered automaticity by the mechanism of *delayed afterdepolarization*.

And each of these mechanisms of arrhythmias can cause disarrangement of the cardiac action, manifesting themselves mostly as ectopic sources of the excitation autowaves. Using new biophysical language, we have attempted to describe below more detailed the currently known types of mechanisms of cardiac arrhythmias.

3.1. Increased automaticity

The term "cardiac automaticity" refers to a biological event characterized by spontaneous process of action potential generation in separate groups of myocardial cells. "Spontaneous" should be understood as being conditioned by intrinsic dynamics, and developing or occurring without apparent external influence, force, cause, or treatment. A spontaneous process is capable of proceeding in a given direction without needing to be driven by an outside source of energy. It is accepted that three different mechanisms may independently underlie cardiac automaticity. These are: (1) the *proper automaticity* of specialized cells of cardiac conduction system, (2) induced automaticity arising or growing under external influences, and (3) triggered activity, which is the automaticity provoked by a series of electrical stimuli.

About the proper automaticity of cardiac conduction system was already told above; it underlies normal cardiac function. It is widely thought that the proper automaticity of specialized myocardiocytes is defined by the capability of cardiac cells to undergo spontaneous diastolic depolarization and to initiate an electrical impulse in the absence of external electrical stimulation. This is so indeed that the specialized conduction system of the heart has the special property of depolarizing without any external influence with a slow, positive increase in voltage across the cell's membrane (the membrane potential) that occurs between the end of one action potential and the beginning of the next action potential. But let's look intently again at Figure 1. Process of spontaneous depolarization corresponds with the motion of the image point from the point D down the left branch of the isoclinic curve $u_t=0$. It is easy to perceive that a self-oscillating element differs from an excitable or from a bistable element only by the absence of the stable steady state at the point **O**. This difference results in birth of a limit cycle[8], which force the element fire again and again. Hence, it is the limit cycle that should be recognized as the cause of the proper automaticity of the specialized myocardiocytes! And what is more, it is likely that a dynamic system described by the base model can be constructed in such manner that the left branch of the isoclinic curve $u_t=0$ would go in the other direction

7 Some people find it difficult to discern the difference between enhanced and increased cardiac automaticity. It seems that to distinguish between enhanced and increased cardiac automaticity is useful for some reasons. While enhanced cardiac automaticity is referred to reactions of normal adaptation (such as influence of autonomic nervous system because of stress), increased cardiac automaticity is addressed rather to pathological alterations of cardiac tissue properties. Some authors prefer using the term "abnormal induced automaticity" instead of "increased cardiac automaticity" (see for example [60]).

8 In mathematics, in the study of dynamical systems with two-dimensional phase space, a limit cycle is a closed trajectory in phase space.

http://dx.doi.org/10.5772/57557

(i.e. line would go from the right top down to the left), and therefore we would have spontaneous diastolic hyperpolarization, — however, a bistable element would fire again and again even in such a case, because of absence of the stable steady state at the point **O** on the left branch. Thus, acceptance of spontaneous diastolic depolarization as a cause of automaticity seems to be a mistake due to misunderstanding of nature of the self-oscillating automaticity.

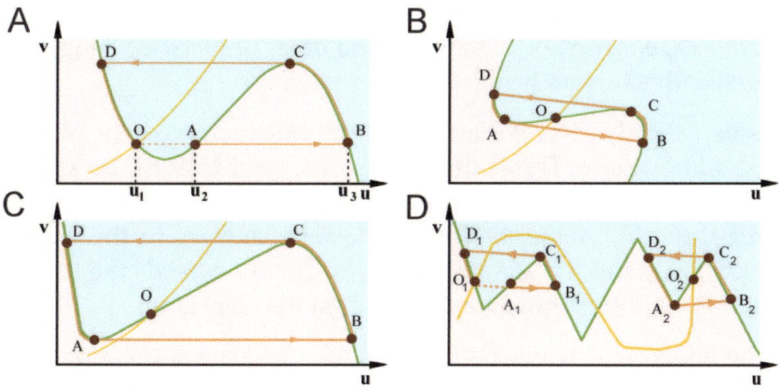

Figure 3. A few examples of increased automaticity caused by transformation of an excitable element in a self-oscillating one. Designations are as in Figure 1. It is assumed that the scale is the same in all examples. See description in the text.

Altered normal automaticity is the proper automaticity of cardiac conduction system altered by certain influences. It should be distinguished between primary and secondary permanent increase of frequency of the self-oscillating elements of cardiac conduction system. While the primary increase is conditioned by the processes that have happened inside the cardiomyocyte, and therefore may be rigid against neural and humoral influences, the secondary increase is caused by the neural and humoral influences, and, consequently, is a reversible process. A classic example of the secondary alteration is hyperthyroidism; myocardial infarction provides with examples of the primary alteration.

Induced automaticity is assumed [41] to result from either transforming a waiting regime of certain myocardial area (or even a single cardiomyocyte) in a self oscillating regime or a sufficient increase of self-oscillating activity of the latent pacemaker cells of the cardiac conduction system. In either case, causes of induced automaticity are similar; among these may be changes of characteristics and ratios of ionic currents in the cell membrane using hormones, poisons, external sources of electric current, etc. Whether the cell spontaneously generates action potential or not, depends on the ratio of incoming and outgoing ion currents. However, as has been stated above, it would be a mistake to assume that it is the spontaneous depolarization after reaching the threshold value of the transmembrane potential that leads to generating spontaneous action potential. Let's look again at Figure 1. The distance between a point of the stable steady state on a branch of the isoclinic curve $u_t = 0$ and the middle section of the same curve (i.e., the segment **OA** in the cases of the excitable regime, as well as the segment $\mathbf{O_1A}$ or $\mathbf{O_2C}$ in the cases of the triggered regime) corresponds with the threshold value; but it is evident, however, that any saying about the threshold value sounds absurdly in the case of the self-oscillating regime because no threshold value exists in this case. The illusion that generating spontaneous action potential is caused by the spontaneous depolarization of cardiac cells has spread widely among physiologists only because of their firm intention to stay strictly within the frames of the mechanistic approach. The real cause of transition of an active element from waiting in a self-oscillating regime is such a deformation of its phase portrait which leads to a shift of the point **O** onto the middle section of the isoclinic curve. Changes of the threshold level also occur as a result of one or another deformation of the phase portrait. Specific causes of the phase portrait deformation are similar in either case; these are again poisons, external electric power sources, and other unpleasant things which are almost certain to disagree with a human being, sooner or later.

Figure 3 gives schematically several examples of the deformation of the phase portrait which leads to induced automaticity. The example D is of special interest, because it assumes that two different attractors exist primordially on the phase portrait.[9] While external stimulus remains near the threshold value, the active element behaves in the waiting regime (the attractor at the left side), but the stimulus that sufficiently exceeds the threshold value will throw it in the self-oscillating regime (the attractor at the right side).

It should only be added that latent pacemakers may become sources of arrhythmias, even when their proper automaticity is maintained on the normal level, but, in the cardiac tissue damaged with disease, a low frequency pacemaker is not synchronized by the waves coming from the sinoatrial node. As a result, the distorted ventricular complexes generated by such a source appear out of turn on the background of normal ECG. Mechanism of such arrhythmia (which is a variant of ventricular extrasystole) could be so-called unidirectional block in a damaged site of myocardium [52], when the autowave excitation is capable of spreading in one direction, but is damped propagating in opposite direction. There may be different causes of such unidirectional block; one of these may be the critical curvature, which was discussed above.

In addition, several autowave objects were described under the general title *"leading centers"* [41, 61–65]. In two-dimensional and three-dimensional excitable media, leading centers emit concentric waves similar to the waves initiated by a pacemaker. At least three different mechanisms of leading centers are known from theoretical studies. One of them is described for media consisting of self-oscillatory elements with hard excitation [62]. Such a medium can be at state of rest (i.e. in the waiting regime), but the place of the medium where an external stimulus of suitable amplitude was applied goes into self-oscillating regime and becomes a source of waves. The two other mechanisms of leading centers were described under the titles of "echo" and "partition of the front." The mechanism "echo" in the myocardium was shown in several works [63–65] with use of microelectrode technique. However, the existence of all these types of autowave sources should still be regarded as hypothetical.

The term *"triggered activity"* (TA) is used to refer to a special kind of automaticity when the cells are in the waiting regime and go into self-oscillating regime in response to a stimulus or series of stimuli. Although differences of opinion still exist, there appears to be good agreement that TA is resulted from *afterdepolarizations*, which is understood as the membrane potential

9 Similar situation in the corresponding phase portrait (i.e. two attractors) is likely to underlie some types of the atrioventricular nodal reentrant tachycardia, which is discussed below.

oscillations that occur during or immediately following a preceding AP (for more details, see [8, 60]). Based on their temporal relationship, two types of afterdepolarizations are described: early afterdepolarizations (EADs), which occur during phase 2 or 3 of the AP, and delayed afterdepolarizations (DADs), which occur after completion of the repolarization phase. There has been increasing recognition of the role played by TA caused by either EADs or DADs in the genesis of clinical arrhythmias [66, 67–69]. It is widely accepted that phenomena of either type of afterdepolarizations are caused by a variety of conditions that raise the diastolic intracellular Ca^{2+} concentration, resulting in Ca^{2+} mediated oscillations that can trigger a new AP if they reach the excitation threshold. It has been found [70] that the active pumping of calcium ions into cardiomyocytes by the Na^+ / Ca^{2+} exchange current of abnormally increased level is involved in the mechanism of DADs. Therefore, the depolarization is observed after treatment of the myocardium with catecholamines [71], which accelerate the pump, as well as with glycosides (e.g., digitalis) [72, 73], which inhibit the Na^+ / K^+ pump, and this leads in turn to the accumulation of intracellular sodium ions and, hence, enhances the intensity of Na^+ / Ca^{2+} pump [74]. Inhibition of the Na^+ / K^+ pump promotes also the release of Ca^{2+} from the sarcoplasmic reticulum, as well as a number of other processes of molecular level are believed to underlie TA [60].

Although the cause of TA is believed to be the transmembrane potential oscillations exceeding the excitation threshold, closer examination of the phase portrait of the basic model is forcing doubt this widespread opinion. As it has already been argued logically above, the excitation threshold can not play any role for self-oscillatory elements, as it simply does not exist in this regime. This fact motivates to search other, more sensible, explanation. Let's assume that the effect of catecholamines and glycosides results in a significant deformation of the phase portrait, and it is the deformation that is the true cause for the change in behavior of the active elements from waiting into a self-oscillating regime, manifesting it in the triggered activity. An important factor in support of this assumption is the following. In the waiting regime, we have a stable solution of node type at the steady point O; a local *bifurcation* of vector fields on the plane occurs while transiting from the waiting regime into the self-oscillating regime, in which the steady point O loses stability, and a new solution, a limit cycle, arises.[10] Thus, in process of the transition of the steady point O from the left branch to the middle section of the isoclinic curve, the system passes through the state, which is referred to as bifurcation; the bifurcation point is situated at the minimum of the N-shaped isocline. Assume that, under the influence of various substances, the null-isocline $f_2(u, v)=0$ moves by parallel displacement along the abscissa from left to right in a linear dependence on the concentration of biologically active substances. What will be observed when the system comes to be near the bifurcation condition? Left from the bifurcation point damped oscillations will be observed, which is in a quite good correspondence with afterdepolarizations without TA. On the right we will observe oscillations with increasing amplitude (the movement by escalating spiral, gradually leading off system onto the right branch of the isocline). In other words, the assumption lead to the conclusion that the base system near the bifurcation point behaves just exactly as it is observed in experiments with TA.

10 The appearance or the disappearance of a periodic orbit through a local change in the stability properties of a steady point is known as the Hopf bifurcation. For more details, see elsewhere [75].

However, the situation may be even more complicated if we consider the phenomena known under the names of "*stability loss delay for dynamical bifurcations*" or "*bifurcation memory*" [19], recently discovered and still little studied. The essence of the effect of bifurcation memory (BM) lies in the appearance of a special, unusual, type of transition process. An ordinary transition process is characterized by asymptotic approach of the dynamical system from the state defined by its initial conditions to the state corresponding to its stable stationary regime in the basin of attraction of which the system found itself. However, near the bifurcation boundary can be observed two types of transition processes. Firstly, passing through the place of the vanished stationary regime, the dynamic system slows down its asymptotic motion temporarily, "*as if recollecting the defunct orbit*" [19]. And only after a number of revolutions of the phase trajectory in this area of bifurcation memory (which is referred to as "*phase spot*"), the phase trajectory rushes to the state that corresponds to stable steady regime for the system. In other words, the decedent attractor still reveals itself in a certain region near the bifurcations, as if it were still "alive", and this strange situation has contributed to appearance of the third name for the phenomena, "*ghost attractor*" [76]. It is possible that the TA is just another example of the bifurcation memory phenomena. It is hoped that new researches will help to clarify the validity of this hypothesis.

Besides, another very specific new mechanism of arrhythmia is assumed [41], which is the so-called *splitting of the excitation wave*. Passing through the damaged area of the heart, the excitation wave may split into two following each other component. Investigation using special blockers has shown that the first component is caused by activation of Na^+-current, and the second is a delayed activation of the Ca^{2+}-current. The auxiliary component, resulting from this splitting, can be a source of extra cardiac beat.

All these autowave phenomena is supposed to be able act as *ectopic foci*, resulting in *ectopic beat* (or cardiac ectopy). Note that nearly all autowave sources mentioned in this section were detected in experiments on myocardium only at very specific experimental conditions. Nevertheless, the physician should bear in mind that the ectopic foci in the myocardium, which gives the characteristic concentric waves of excitation, can be not only an unregulated latent pacemaker. This remark is entirely correct also regarding so-called *polytopic tachycardias*, which may be based on essentially different mechanisms of ectopia.

3.2. Circulating autowaves (reentry)

The concept of circulation of the excitation wave, which is so important for understanding the mechanisms of a number of types of high-frequency cardiac arrhythmias (tachycardias), has been confirmed experimentally in 1926 by D. Scherf and C. Schockhoff [8], and now it is widely recognized that the circulation of excitation (reentry) is not confined within conducting tissues, but can occur in any region of the heart.

3.3. A single two-dimensional autowave vortex

It is known that reentrant cardiac arrhythmias are often initiated by forming a discontinuous propagating wave of excitation. In sufficiently thin layers (i.e., in two-dimensional media, in mathematical language), it is refractoriness that makes possible the existence of special *circulating autowaves* (Figure 4), which evolve from wave fronts with the free tip originating from rupture of the wave front. In a thin layer of active medium of sufficiently large extent ("infinite" from the point of view of mathematics, i.e. a layer of such extent when a further increase in the size does not affect the behavior of the object under study), the rotating autowaves take shape of rotating spirals. It was shown already in the axiomatic models of Wiener-Rosenbluth [40] that the discontinuity of a plane wave of excitation, which results from its collision with a sufficiently large non-excitable obstacle, makes the excitation wave revolve around this obstacle. Further studies have shown that the availability of obstacles is not required without fail and that the rotating autowaves also arises when creating the appropriate initial conditions. For example, the inhomogeneity of tissue refractoriness may lead to the fact that at high repetition frequency of the excitation waves the wave front may break on roughness of the tail of the preceding wave, and the evolution of these ruptures leads to the formation of rotating autowaves.

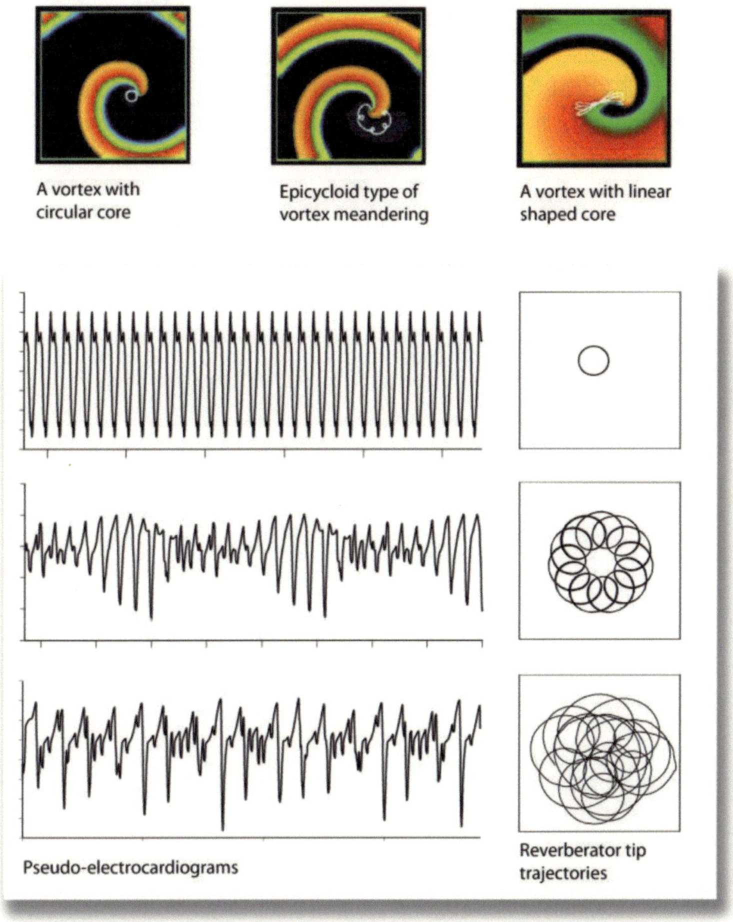

Figure 4. Some classic types of reverberator evolution. The inset demonstrates examples of ECG forms for different types of evolution of reverberator: uniform circular rotation (top), meander (middle), and hyper-meander (bottom).

It is customary to distinguish four variants of circulating autowaves (see [8, 41], for example):

1. The *spiral wave*, which is an excitation autowave *revolving around an obstacle*. An example of this is atrial flutter due to the autowave moving around cardiac veins.

2. The *autowave running around the ring* (synonym: one-dimensional circulation regime). Examples of arrhythmias caused by such type of reentry are: (1) the excitation wave circulation between the atria and ventricles through additional atrioventricular path during tachycardia associated with WPW-syndrome; (2) supraventricular tachycardia caused by the excitation wave circulation in the AV node; (3) intraventricular circulations of the excitation wave along path consisting of the specialized cardiac conduction system.

3. The autowave *reverberator*, which is two-dimensional circulation of autowave with its free tip in the plane of the heart wall in the area of myocardium without anatomic obstacle (i.e., *two-dimensional autowave vortex*). In contrast to the circulation around the obstacle, the position of the center of this type of circulating autowaves in this case can move through the cardiac tissue (i.e., it can drift) during arrhythmia. With use of both the multielectrode and optical mapping the existence of such sources of arrhythmias in real myocardium was demonstrated in the SA node as well as in the atrial and ventricular cardiac tissue.

4. Autowave *fibrillation*, which is chaotic regime of autowave propagation.

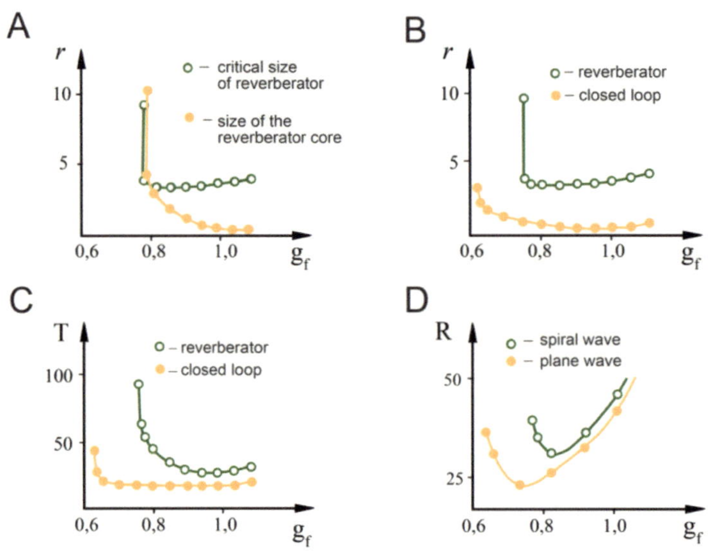

Figure 5. The critical size of reverberator (based on data from [41] obtained by Pertsov and Panfilov for the FitzHugh-Nagumo model). **A**. The relation between the critical size of reverberator and the size of the reverberator core. **B**. The dependences of the critical sizes of reverberator and of the critical size of a closed loop (for an autowave running around the ring) on the conduction of rapid current g_f. **C**. Dependences of the period of the reverberator and of the autowave running around the ring on g_f. **D**. Dependence of the refractoriness of the medium (*R*) on g_f for the spiral wave (curvature *k*=0.83) and for the plane wave.

It is necessary to pay attention to some of the subtleties of terminology. Various authors can refer to the rotating in two-dimensional medium autowave as "spiral wave", "reverberator", "rotor", "autowave vortex" or even "scroll wave". Note, however, that these terms are not interchangeable synonymous. Briefly, there are the following differences between them. The term "spiral wave" refers usually only to the autowave that revolves around non-excitable obstacle in a medium of sufficiently large extent, that is, in this case, the medium of such size, comparing with which the obstacle is small, but large enough to result in the wave break. The tip of the spiral wave moves along the boundary of the non- excitable obstacle. The authors of [41] pointed out: "The most important difference between a reverberator and a spiral wave rotating around the hole, which is similar to reverberator in its form, is that the reverberator is not tied to any structure in the medium. Due to this property, reverberators can appear and disappear at different locations of the medium." Moreover, the autowave reverberators have property to appear not only in the absence of non-excitable obstacles, but also in a completely homogeneous medium (under appropriate initial conditions).

Furthermore, it proved (Figure 5) that refractory period is longer for waves with nonzero curvature (i.e., for reverberators) than for a plane autowave (i.e., the autowave running around the ring), and refractory period of reverberators begins to increase before increase of refractory period of a plane wave, when the excitability of the medium decreases. These and other significant differences of reverberator from circular movement of the excitation wave make us distinguish between these two regimes of reentry.

In the simplest case without drift (i.e., the regime of *uniform circular rotation*), the tip of a reverberator rotates around a fixed point along the circumference of a certain radius (the circular motion of the tip of the reverberator). The autowave cannot penetrate into the circle bounded by this circumference. As far as it approaches the centre of the reverberator rotation, the amplitude of the excitation pulse is reduced, and, at a relatively low excitability of the medium there is a region of finite size in the centre of reverberator, where the amplitude of the excitation pulse is zero (recall that we speak now about a homogeneous medium, for each point of which its properties are the same). This area of low amplitude in the centre of the reverberator is usually called the *core of the reverberator*. The existence of such a region in the center of reverberator seems, at first glance, quite incomprehensible, as it borders all the time with the excited sites. A detailed investigation of this phenomenon showed [41] that resting area in the centre of reverberator remains of its normal excitability, and the existence of a quiescent region in the centre of the reverberator is related to the phenomenon of the critical curvature. In the case of "infinite" homogeneous medium, the core radius and the speed of the rotor rotation are determined only by the properties of the medium itself, rather than the initial conditions. The certain size of the core of the reverberator is conditioned by that the excitation wave, which circulates in a closed path, should completely fit in this path without bumping into its own refractory tail.

The *critical size of reverberator* is understood as the minimum size of the active homogeneous medium in which the reverberator can exist during indefinitely long time. To assess the critical size of reverberator, some authors (e.g., [61]) used the size of the core of the reverberator, supposing that the region of the medium that is adjacent to the core is sufficient for the existence of sustainable reentry. However, accurate quantitative study of the dependence of the reverberator behavior on conductivity of rapid transmembrane current (which characterizes the excitability of the medium) has revealed [41] that the critical size and the size of the reverberator core are its different characteristics (Figure 5), and the critical size of reverberator is, in many cases, much larger than the size of its core (i.e., reverberator perishes even when its core easily fit within the boundaries of the medium and its drift is absent). It was shown also that, for the same local characteristics of an excitable medium (excitability, refractoriness, etc. given by the nonlinear free member of the base model), there are significant quantitative differences in dependencies of characteristics of the reverberator and of one-dimensional circulation of the autowave impulse, although corresponding curves coincide qualitatively. It is assumed that the earlier growth of the refractory period and of the critical size of reverberator with a decrease of excitability is caused by the curvature of the wavefront of reverberator.

The one-dimensional circulation regime, which is perhaps the simplest case of circulating autowaves, has been studied in greatest detail, and the results help to understand more intricate variants of reentry. In particular, it was shown [55] that the existence of this type of reentry is only possible on condition that the size of the closed loop in which the circulation occurs is greater than a minimal size (the *critical size of the closed loop*). Size of *the core of the reverberator* is usually less than the *critical size of the closed loop* for circular movement, which is associated with the phenomenon of *critical curvature* (Figure 5). Note that, in the normal myocardium (i.e., with normal velocity of excitation autowave, $V \approx 1$ m / sec, and with normal refractory period, $R \approx 0{,}2$ sec), the wavelength ($V = R\,\lambda$) is about 20 centimeters, and, therefore, it is difficult, even nearly impossible, for circulating wave to fit in the human heart, if there are not any special conditions. Probability of arising of reverberator in the human heart under normal state of the myocardium is small, but the decreases of refractory period or of the excitation wave velocity (under the influence of metabolism, under the pharmacological influence, etc.) contribute to the appearance of circulating waves in the myocardium.

A reverberator is able to drift freely in medium; besides direction of its drift is caused not only by the properties of the medium, but also largely by its own properties (i.e., the reverberator itself "decides" where to move). In the classical works [32, 42, 77], the following basic types of reverberator behavior in a homogeneous isotropic medium (Figure 4) are distinguished: (1) the regime of *uniform circular rotation* (circular movement), which is the simplest case without drift, with the tip of a reverberator rotating around a fixed point along the circumference of a certain radius; (2) *meander*, which is two-periodic motion of the reverberator in which the trajectory of its tip is similar to a cycloidal curve (epicycloid and hypocycloid); (3) *hyper-meander*, which is a complicated reverberator motion with, probably, chaotic trajectory of its tip. Under special conditions, a vortex with meandering of hypocycloid type can be transformed to a vortex with *linear core* [77].

Recently a new form of autowave behavior was found [21], — namely, the transformation of reverberator motion from a two-periodic meander into one-periodic circular rotation due to spontaneous deceleration of reverberator drift. The new autowave behavior, which was called "*autowave lacet*", is likely to result from a phenomenon of so called bifurcation memory. When autowave lacet was discovered, the first question arose: Does the meander exist ever or the halt of the reverberator drift can be observed every time in all the cases, which are called meander, if the observation will be sufficiently long? The comparative quantitative analysis of the drift velocity of reverberator in the regimes of meander and lacet revealed a clear difference between these two types of evolution of the reverberator: while the drift velocity quickly goes to a stationary value during meander, a steady decrease in the drift velocity of the vortex can be observed during the lacet, in which can be clearly identified the phase of slow deceleration and phase of rapid deceleration of the drift velocity.

The revealing of autowave lacet may be important for cardiology, because the autowave theory predicts the existence of special type of ventricular arrhythmias, conditionally called *"lacetic"* [1, 2], which cardiologists do not still distinguish in diagnostics.

When an autowave propagates in a medium and collides with an obstacle containing a slit, propagation beyond the slit depends on the relationship between the width of the slit and the liminal region. When the slit dimensions are greater than the liminal region, then the wave fragment passing through the slit will continue to propagate. In addition, the ends of the newly formed wave fragment will curl and form counter-rotating autowave vortices, which can results in cardiac tachycardia or fibrillation. [47].

Even more interesting phenomenon caused by the critical curvature effects is *unidirectional conduction* of excitation autowave through a narrow gap in a non-excitable partition arising in the case if the partition edges are arranged at an angle to one another [52].

Variety of forms of behavior of autowave vortices leads to the variety of cardiac arrhythmias, which can be quite ambiguous reflected in the electrocardiograms [1].

At this point, this brief overview of two-dimensional circulating autowaves must be stopped, and more detailed information about their multifarious behavior can be found in the extensive literature.

3.4. Three-dimensional autowave vortices

Even more intricate types of reentry arise "in the three-dimensional case", in the parlance of mathematicians [13, 78–80]. Figure 6 gives examples of three-dimensional organization of reentrant propagation. Direct generalization of an autowave reverberator for the case of three-dimensional space is a *simple scroll*, which rotation occurs around a straight line, called *"filament"*. In addition to such a simple three-dimensional autowave reentry, the filament can be arbitrarily curved and possibly even closed (in the latter case, the scroll turns into an *autowave scroll ring*). If the rotational phase of the scroll varies along its filament, the vortex is called *"twisted scroll"*. Despite the much greater variety of three-dimensional autowave regimes in comparison with two-dimensional case, it was mathematically proven that there are certain topological restrictions, which reduce significantly the variety of three-dimensional autowave structures. For example, a single twisted scroll ring is impossible; topologically there must be another filament passing through the center of the filament ring [81].

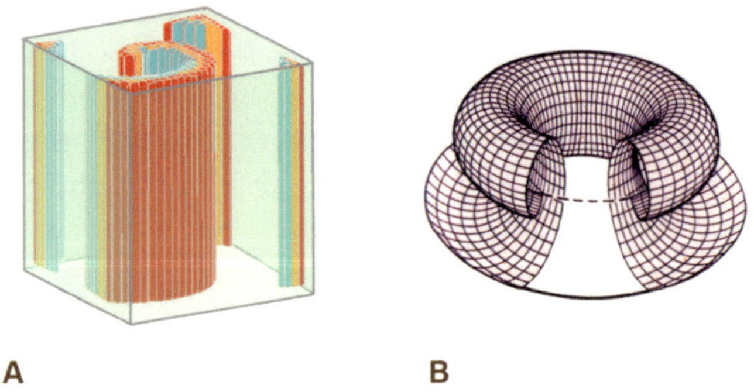

Figure 6. Examples of autowave 3D-vortices: **A** — a simple scroll, **B** — a simple vortex ring.

Although the scroll filament is a bit of a virtual object, it was shown [79] that it has a special property, which has been called *tension* of filaments. A filament with positive tension tends to shorten, similar to an elastic band, and, for example, the autowave scroll ring "shrinks" as a result. When being with negative tension, it increases in size, which eventually ends in multiple twisting of the filament, in its ruptures and in total chaotization of the autowave behavior, — and it looks like ventricular fibrillation (inasmuch as the atrial walls are much thinner, an intricate autowave three-dimensional structure cannot be placed there). The reader should give attention to the fact that the filament tension is a phenomenon caused by the properties of the active medium, and not by the properties of the autowave vortex arising in this medium.

A new mechanism of stabilizing the motion of an autowave vortex was described in the same work for the case of three-dimensional excitable medium with a positive tension of filament; the stabilization occurs due to shortening of the filament attached to the transverse walls of model media. Although ECG manifestations of such stabilization of a vortex motion are not considered in [79], the obvious conclusion in this case is that there would be observed a spontaneous transition of tachycardia from polymorphic to monomorphic type. Thus, stabilization of an autowave three-dimensional vortex with positive tension due to shortening its filament is today the third possible mechanism of such electrocardiographic transformation (the two others are anchoring the autowave vortex in an obstacle and tachycardia of the lacetic type [1]). Note that the anchoring and the lacetic tachycardia are still hypothetical, and their detection in real myocardium requires further research.

3.5. Multiple reverberators and autowave fibrillation

One of the most important results of the study of autowave processes is disclosure of a new mechanism of instability in the active media [30, 42] associated with reproduction of reverberators. As mentioned earlier, wave-fronts sent by reverberator follow closely to each other, and therefore a subsequent wave-front may be broken on the irregularities of the tail of the previous wave-front. It is recognized that (1) reverberators cannot reproduce themselves in a homogeneous medium, and (2) the waves give rise to a new reverberator in an inhomogeneous medium only if the period of these waves is sufficiently small (roughly equal to the relative refractory period). The latter circumstance is used in physiological experiments to provoke tachycardia: two consecutive pulses are sent through the stimulating electrode, and if the second pulse falls within the "window of vulnerability" (i.e., at the time of relative refractoriness), then an experimental reentrant arrhythmia occurs [34]. It is also assumed that a similar mechanism (collision of an extra wave of excitation to the refractory tail of the previous wave) underlies clinical paroxysmal tachycardias, such as atrial flutter, paroxysmal supraventricular or ventricular tachycardia [8].

It was shown in theoretical studies with use of axiomatic models [41] that another significant property of the reverberator is a finite time of his life in heterogeneous environments. Causes of destruction of reverberator are the same as the causes for its rise, and consist in the inability of steady propagation of excitation waves with high frequency in heterogeneous media. These conclusions are well confirmed in experiments: a reverberator in a homogeneous chemical medium has "infinite" lifetime (limited by depletion of reagents), but in the heart, where there is large heterogeneity, an arising accidentally reverberator usually have time to send only a few wave-fronts.

Thus, there are two competing processes in an inhomogeneous medium: reproduction of reverberators and their death. When the reproduction rate is less than the rate of death, then chaos is impossible, and the medium works in regular mode. In the opposite case, the number of autowave sources begins to grow, leading to chaos. This process reproduces well all main phenomena observed in the heart during fibrillation [41, 42]. Here, similar to the phenomenon of critical mass in the chain reactions, some critical characteristic values appear, above which there is an unlimited reproduction of reverberators. One of these characteristics is the so-called *critical mass of fibrillation*, which is the minimum mass of cardiac tissue, above which fibrillation becomes possible.

The historically first point of view on ventricular fibrillation was that it is a passive process: the jaded heart cannot longer conduct the excitation through the myocardium and only a few Purkinje fibers, after losing control from the pacemaker of higher hierarchy, continue spontaneously to cause asynchronous excitation of myocardial fibers. Currently, though multifocal ectopic activity of ventricular myocardium remains still being considered as a possible mechanism of fibrillation, the main mechanism of ventricular fibrillation is widely recognized to be reentry within the ventricles, which may occur for one cause or another [7, 8, 60,]. Development of ideas about myocardium as an active medium led to significantly different views on the nature of ventricular fibrillation. For example, it has been shown that the ECG that is typical for ventricular fibrillation can be observed resulting from at least two different autowave mechanisms: as a result of coexistence multiple autowave vortices or of a single vortex due to Wenckebach-like frequency division, which in turn is due to some peculiarities inhomogeneity of the active medium [80].

However, such an interesting hypothesis about the nature of ventricular fibrillation as a competing chain reactions of birth and death of reverberators is not received still the merited popularity among researchers and remains without its further development. It is hoped that new researches will give a new development for this hypothesis.

4. Basic mechanisms of adaptation and their abnormalities

Earlier in this chapter we have attempted to show how significantly opportunities of researchers in the interpretation of various phenomena of cardiac action were expanded with using biophysical language, which constitutes a substantial generalization of the experience of two centuries of studies of the heart. But it must be also recognized that the cybernetic language, the basis of which was provided by Norbert Wiener in his classic work [82], is equally useful generalization for aims of cardiology. This section of the chapter is intended for outlining the fundamental cybernetic ideas about the cardiac action and its disorders, with the subsequent text based mainly on Fedorov's[11] work [83], which is scarcely known for English readers.

In the tradition of biophysics, the regulation of heart rate is modeled in isolation; in other words, the heart is assumed to be an autonomous organ, in which its own rhythmic contraction is determined by spontaneous activity of the sinus node myocardiocytes (as it was described above in this chapter), although it is assumed a number of both humoral and neural factors that can modulate this spontaneous activity. In contrast to the pure biophysical approach, cyberneticists used to simulate the regulation of cardiac rhythm as a part of certain regulatory circuits in a more general model of the cardiovascular system rather than isolated.[12] Biological systems contain many types of regulatory circuits, both positive and negative; and construction of a scheme of regulatory circuits, i.e. a typical for traditional physiology descriptive model of regulation, is certainly based on considerations about purpose of functioning of a mechanism or a system that is under studying. Instead the word "purpose", the fixed expression "*physiological role*" (of the system or of the mechanism) is accepted to use in biological sources, the term "*target function*" corresponding with it in the frames of the cybernetic approach.

It is recognized that the most important purpose of functioning of the blood circulatory system (including also external respiration), i.e. the most important "physiological role" of the blood circulation, is the timely delivery of oxygen, nutritious and other substances to all the cells of the body, as well as removal of accumulated metabolites and heat from the tissues; and this ensures maintenance of the internal environment, which surrounds the cells and is necessary for implementation of their metabolism and their biological functions. Open- and closed-loop control as well as a good number of guidance loops is involved in the *inherent regulation* [13] of circulation. It is accepted that the inherent circulatory regulation includes all changes in the cardiovascular system which are directed to preventing or reducing every threatening alteration of the internal environment and metabolism of cells. Consideration of separate mechanisms of the inherent circulatory regulation reveals that the regulation provides it also with achieving an additional goal, which is maintenance of the blood circulation as itself and economization of the blood flow reserve. This substantiates the assignment of the cardiovascular apparatus to the category of a separate functional system of the organism. Besides the

---

11 Viktor FedorovichFedorov carried out this investigation during his work on PhD thesis on the base of the Department of Telemedicine of Medical Center attached to the Presidential Property Management Directorate.

12 By the way, this is one of the reasons why the modern "cardiophysics" is not synonymous with the modern "cardiovascular biophysics".

13 In the original [83]:«автоматическое управление кровообращением».

tasks of control of maintaining the internal environment at the chosen level, the biological inherent regulation includes also mechanisms of self-adjustment (*adaptation*) of the control systems in accordance with changes in the parameters of the biological object or of external influences, as well as mechanisms of automatic selection of the best modes. In view of this the broader term "*inherent guidance*" (or "*self-guidance*") is believed to be more appropriate to describe the functioning of living systems. It should be noted that a human being is characterized with a very complex mental activity; on this occasion, P.K Anokhin, a famous Russian physiologist who developed the theory of functional systems [84, 85], pointed out a significant influence of motivation and memory on the result of afferent synthesis, i.e. not physical, but purely informational in its nature stimuli are important for results of inherent circulatory regulation. Hence, the sinus rhythm of the human heart reflects the work of many body systems in normal and pathological conditions, and therefore it is quite reasonable to recognize the possibility of making use of its parameters for constructing a quantitative measure of the quality of individual health.

However, we must here pay attention to the paradoxical situation existing in theoretical medicine today, when any disease (except for the most exotic) is fully described and classified by its stages as well as is easily scaled by its severity, but at the same time a scaling (a set of standardized quantitative measures of the quality) of health is absent, although people widely use in everyday life words of comparing people's health.

According to the new conception of measuring human health [86] that was developed at the Department of Medical and Biological Cybernetics of the Russian State Medical University (Moscow) and was approved by Russian Ministry of Health about two decades ago, the health is understood as "*the system's ability to achieve its aims through its adequate behavior*". Analysis of the ultimate goals of the diverse forms of behavior of living systems can reduce all of these goals to two aims, which are self-reproduction and self-preservation (and keen rivalry between them in the nature is usually resolved in favor of the first). The main idea which was advanced in this connection is to make "*an assessment of individual health or social health (health of a population) on the base of the ability of the living systems to self-development, to self-preservation, to reproduction of offspring as well as to reproduction of the means for implementation of their goals and adequate forms of their behavior*". In the same paradigm, adequate forms of behavior of living systems are grouped as follows:

- self-organization, understood as ability of the system to implement process of dynamic structural and functional self-development with differentiation of some collections of elements for a function;
- adaptability, i.e. the system's ability to adjust itself to changing environmental conditions while retaining its identity and its main functional properties;
- active transformation of the environment (i.e., natural habitat) as a form of adaptation, consequences for the social system should be to create harmony of the noosphere (according to V.I. Vernadsky).

It is easy to see in this construction that self-organization, and active habitat transformation is based on adaptive properties, which are typical for all living things.

In this regard, it is extremely important to remember that adaptive properties of a natural living system is aimed at survival of the biological population[14] as a whole rather than to survival of the single individual in the population, which is conditioned by the process of biological evolution (for instance, by means of natural selection). P.V. Simonov, another illustrious Russian physiologist, has written [87] on this subject: "*mechanism of myocardial infarction has been formed already in the evolution of the relict salmon. As a working hypothesis, we tend to consider cardiovascular pathology of neurogenic origin as a result of a long evolution of one of the mechanisms that enforce the stability and qualitative improvement of the population through the elimination of those individuals that adapts poorly in certain conditions of the existence of our distant ancestors. (...) Since passive animals are often better protected from external dangers (predators, traps, etc.) than individuals with active-searching behavior, natural selection could lead to the accumulation of passive cowards in the population, which would denote regression of the species while increasing its sustainability. This risk of degeneration seems to have been eliminated by means of genetic linkage between the tendency to passive-defensive behavior and susceptibility to cardiovascular and some other psychosomatic diseases. An extreme but striking example of such behavior is suicidal tendency among the subjects with chronic depressive syndrome.*" It seems that the recent investigations [88] prove such conclusions. Despite the fact that this context generates a number of ethical issues, which are known as moral dilemmas[15], any ignoring of such biological mechanisms would be a huge mistake.

In the adaptive responses of a biological system (an organism), it is useful to distinguish the ability to implement the process of adaptation, the process itself and its result. Therefore, with respect to adaptive reactions of a human individual, from our point of view, we can formulate the following definitions. *Adaptation* of a human is the process of such adjusting changes of the organism and of the personality under the influence of totality of conditions of habitat that provide an approximation to the optimal values of the efficiency and reliability of implementation of adequate patterns of human behavior. *Adaptedness* is understood as the state of having been adapted, which is also the measure the current result of adaptation. *Adaptability* is the measure that reflects the ability of a biological system to change its adaptedness per unit of time.

Practical experience shows that a high level of adaptedness to certain specific conditions (i.e., high specialization) leads to a loss of adaptability (universality), and vice versa. Consequently, either extreme reduces the reliability of functioning of the organism. On the basis of these theses an individual human health can be defined as follows.

Individual health is a measure that expresses the ratio between adaptedness and adaptability of the individual. At that, the optimal state of health should be understood as a state of satisfactory adaptedness to the specific conditions of the individual existence while maintaining sufficient adaptability (adaptive readiness to a sudden change of conditions).

---

14 A biological species can be considered as a set (in the mathematical meaning) of consanguineous (closely-related) biological populations.

15 In-depth analysis of moral dilemmas was given in [89] recently, so we will not dwell on this issue here.We should only note that similar problems are encountered when finding the optimal balance between the values of the unity of a nation and the values of liberal freedoms.

Consequently, the character of the deviations in the action of the heart from its normal action must be considered from the standpoint of assessment of deviations in state of a human from his or her optimal state of health. How this should be done?

When considering a practically healthy person with the saved in varying degrees adaptive mechanisms, the process of adaptation to functioning in conditions of permissible physical or mental exertion is taking the form of a quasi-linear increase of the corresponding function with an increase in exertion. The linear dependence in coordinates of "stress-response" is broken only in the areas of imperceptible (i.e., while having a subthreshold level of stress) or extreme exertions (i.e., when exhaustion of the reserve of adaptation occurs). In other words, the whole curve "stress-response" reveals a sort of S-shaped dependence (i.e., the logistic sigmoid function). There are five sites that can be identified on this curve (Figure 7). It is obvious that the nature of the load as well as parameters of response may vary in description of the different systems or organs of the human body. It may be a special load, which has an influence only on a number of certain parameters of the organism (e.g., the influence of illumination on the pupil diameter), or a sort of universal load, in response to which the parameters of all or most of the organs and the systems become changed (such as hypoxia). The response parameters need not be primary (measured directly). As those, in some cases, one may make use of the results of mathematical processing of time series of individual primary parameters or even different mathematical combinations of several primary parameters that characterize a particular function of the body. The main requirement for the choice of such parameters is that each parameter showing the response of the organism should change with increasing load like the logistic function and should conform to physiological functions.

It is obvious that the various organs and systems of the body are not necessarily to be in the same functional state. So the pathology of certain organs or systems may result in not only functional, but also structural change of other organs for compensating the reduced function. Therefore, to describe the whole organism by the proposed method, it is required to develop a system of tests that assess separate responses of different organs and systems on a load which is typical for each of them. A specific component of quantitative assessment of the health quality of a particular person can be obtained by making comparison of the slope and the level of saturation of the logistic curve, which corresponds to the response on an adequate load, in a specific plane, which conforms with a specific organ or a specific system, with the average statistical parameters of healthy individuals of the corresponding sex and age group. A set of such "response-planes", each of these with its own parameters (A, B, C, D), enables us to build a system of quantitative assessment of the quality of individual health. By tracking the dynamics of change of the parameters of the curves in each plane simultaneously, we can assess the level of total individual health.

The medical examination should be fulfilled as a three-phase test, comprising the successive phases: 1) initial phase of rest, 2) phase of the individually metered load, and 3) recovery phase. This is caused by the following circumstances.

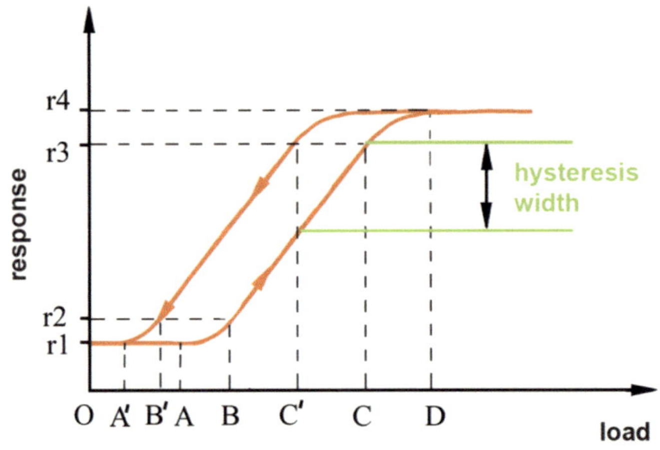

Figure 7. Typical response curves obtained during the testing process with linear increase and subsequent linear decrease of load. Five sections can be identified on each curve: **OA** — the zone of areactivity, when the load is so small that the response is inexpedient; **AB** — the initial nonlinear part of the response, when the specific reaction grows with load increases (can be approximated by a power or exponential functions); **BC** — the zone of linear regulation, when the reaction increase is proportional to the load growth; **CD** — the final non-linear section, when the responding system is approaching exhaustion of resources for adaptation; the section right of **D** corresponds with resource exhaustion response. Arrows show the direction of the process. The projection of the distance between linear sections of the load curve (ascending part of the loop) and the recovery curve (its descending part) on the axis of reactions is taken as the "*width of the hysteresis loop*".

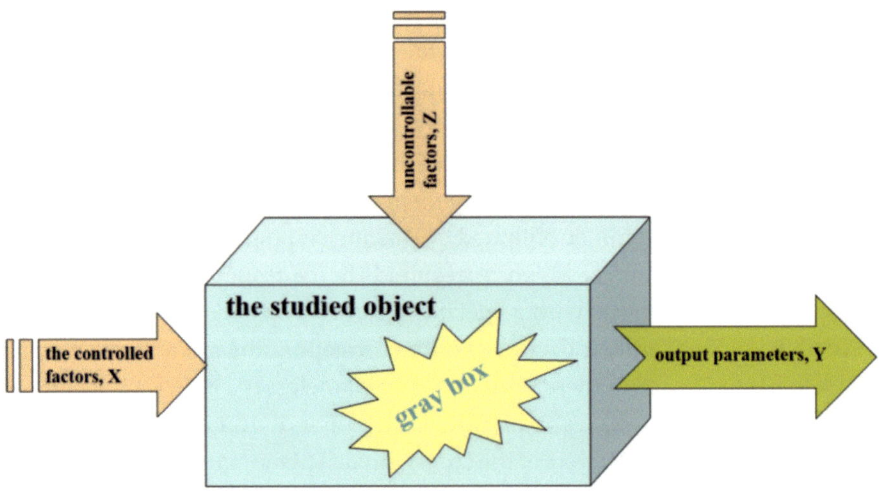

Figure 8. The general scheme of the two approaches (black and gray boxes). **X** — vector of input influences; **Y** — vector of output measured parameters; **Z** — vector uncontrolled influences.

When investigating the complex system (and many researchers are inclined to reckon human organism among supercomplex systems) about the internal structure of which is not known everything that is required to know for predicting its behavior under different conditions, the approaches of "black box" or of "gray box" (Figure 8) are taken to use in cybernetics. Either approach provides for an impact on the studied object by a number of certain controllable factors (the vector of the input parameters) with subsequent registration of the vector of the output parameters. While changing the quantitative levels of the input vector or composition of these parameters, one can observe some changes of the output vector with the aim to find out the transition function, which is inherent in the object under study. In general, we can write the expression $\vec{Y} = F(\vec{X}, \vec{Z})$, i.e. the output parameters are a function of both the input (controlled) impacts and a complex of uncontrolled influences. In our particular case, a doctor or a researcher has a number of certain ideas about the form of the function (or more precisely, a set of models that approximately describe it); in other words, our box is "gray", not "black". However, even when the form of the function F is known exactly, but we do not know anything about the vector $\vec{Z}$, the correct prediction of how the system behavior changes with changing the vector $\vec{X}$ can scarcely be done. As long as the task of a detailed description of the vector $\vec{Z}$, seems to be unsolvable in principle when the cardiovascular system is under the study (since, for example, emotionally significant reflections of the patient have a significant effect on the cardiac rhythm as well as on blood pressure, but they cannot be put under an external control), the only way to solve the problem of revealing the transition function is the way of shifting the conditions of studying the cardiac action to the situation that can be described by the inequality $\vec{X} >> \vec{Z}$(in the appropriate meaning). To reach the situation, one can either transfer some of the factors from the $\vec{Z}$ to the $\vec{X}$ (if it is possible), or raise the components of the vector $\vec{X}$ to such values when the control system of the biological object being studied will be forced to neglect the influence of $\vec{Z}$ for reasons of self-preservation.

Hence, the testing of a complex system the sufficient information about which is not available should be carried out under the influence of a set of controlled factors (the load) the total effect of which is much higher than that of the unrecorded influences. In other words, the medical examination of the cardiac action should always be performed with the phase of such level of the individually metered load that is physiologically significant for the organism of the examined individual.

No matter how little the test influence is applied, the cardiovascular system, as well as the organism as a whole, functions in a "background mode" nevertheless, in accordance with a great number of the natural laws. So the information about the level of functioning of the organism at rest (at below-threshold loads) is also required, and, therefore, every part of the dependence in coordinates of "stress-response" provides some useful information about the organism.

After canceling any significant load, the system can not instantly jump to its original state because of its inertial properties associated primarily with changes in concentrations of various substances (both hormones and metabolites) in response to the foregoing load. For bringing the substances to their initial concentration, their diffusion, transport and metabolism require some time and energy costs. Hence, the recovery process contains not less information about the system than its actual response to the load. To assess the response of the load, one of the most convenient models is that one in which a linear increase of load up to a predetermined level followed by a linear decline of load to zero (for example, using veloergometry) is implemented. Curves obtained in this way are reminiscent of the hysteresis loop in descriptions of the magnetization reversal of ferromagnets with high coercivity. The curves from tests with increasing load to a submaximal level have the form shown in Figure 7. The width of the hysteresis loop in this case reflects the adaptability of the reacting system.

The basic mechanisms of cardiovascular regulation, as well as methods for assessing their integrity in the cases when spatial-temporal organization of the heart remains near normality, have been described briefly in this section of the chapter. In such cases, the methods recommended will help more effectively identify persons with weakened adaptive ability at maintenance of normal heart functioning. According to the well-known joke, "healthy people do not exist, there are only people that did still not get the sufficiently full checkup"; and it looks like a great truth.

5. Conclusion: Arrhythmic action of the heart

It has been believed for centuries that cardiac arrhythmia is a sort of pathology, excepting a few variants, caused by these or those disorders of cardiac activity. However, the facts that is set out in this chapter make us become engrossed in our thoughts about many cases when arrhythmia may be a specific sort of normal activity of the heart (and the cardiovascular system in whole), which should be regarded as a normal adaptive response of an organism either on some other health problems, which are different from cardiac problem, or on some specific external signals. And medical treatment in either situation seems to be harmful, and accordingly increases the overall mortality rate from treated cases of arrhythmia (the problem that was addressed in the beginning of the chapter).

In some cases, it has the character of a reversible adaptive response, in other cases it is a compensatory response aimed at replacement of certain lost functions of the organism, and all such cases should be taken as a *normal arrhythmic functioning of the heart*. Certain types of arrhythmias are dangerous to life of the whole organism, because they call forth hemodynamic disturbances, which in turn lead to dysfunction of various vital organs. This group of arrhythmias includes also those that are started up by certain natural hereditary mechanisms of the population dynamics regulation, which should also be recognized, from the viewpoint of the biomedical sciences, as a sort of the normal arrhythmic functioning of the heart. Recall that, according to the hypothesis expressed by P.K Anokhin, even myocardial infarction, at least in some cases, should be considered as a specific adaptive reaction realized through certain mechanisms of intra-population self-regulation. Developing Anokhin's hypothesis, we propose a new special term *"arrhythmic action of the heart"*, which should be comprehended as the normal arrhythmic functioning of the heart that is aimed at maintenance of physiological homeostasis under certain specific conditions.

In some other cases, we are often faced with *pathological arrhythmic functioning of the heart*, of course. Therefore, the actual problem of modern medicine is the development of objective methods for discerning arrhythmic action of the heart and *arrhythmic disorders of the action of the heart*

Note that the evaluation of serious cardiac arrhythmias associated with the change in location of the source of excitation waves is even more difficult. For example, the case reported previously [1] engenders thoughts that even the atrioventricular nodal reentrant tachycardia (AVNRT) should be considered in the certain cases as a variant of the normal adaptive response. To observe and to study the normal variants of the AVNRT is harder for two obvious reasons. Firstly, when a human is moving very actively, taking measurements of his or her physiological parameters becomes a very difficult task. Secondly, there are a relatively small number of people in populations of modern societies, who are able to undergo very high physical loads. But it must be assumed that in ancient times, when living conditions were much more rigorous, the normal type of AVNRT could play a vitally important role in providing physiological needs of an actively moving human (during an extremely quick run, for example). It is reasonable to assume that the biological evolution has given our ancestors this normal type of AVNRT as a reserve mechanism for increasing cardiac rate during extremely high physical loads, when it is needed more frequent rhythm of cardiac contraction than the highest possible rhythm of the sinoatrial node. If this hypothesis will be confirmed, clinical cases of AVNRT should be seen rather as a disease resulting from decrease of control from the side of the functional system that regulates the cardiac action, than as pathology of the atrioventricular node.

Another important point is concerned with the widespread conception in the medical community that the arrhythmia must be understood as some abnormalities in the electrical activity of the heart or in conduction of excitation waves through the myocardium. Under this conception, disturbance of other cardiac functions, such as the contractile function, does not relate to cardiac arrhythmias, although can result in arrhythmia of this or that type. This understanding of cardiac arrhythmia is based on traditional rough notions of cause-and-effect relations between processes that underlie the cardiac action. It is traditionally accepted that the process of excitation of the membranes of cardiomyocytes causes contraction of these cells, which in turn leads to the ejection of blood from the heart. Everything here is seems to be simple, logical and understandable, but...

Recent studies [90–92] have demonstrated that the nature in this case also proved to be "smarter" than the human logic built within the frames of the mechanistic approach. The new experimental results reveal the existence of negative feedback, in the terms of cybernetics, between the contractile function of the heart and the process of its electrical excitation, as well as the substantial effect of the mechanical conditions of cardiac contraction on the process of cardiac excitation. In contrast to the rather well-studied nature of the coupling between excitation and contraction, the molecular-cellular mechanisms of *mechanoelectrical feedback* and its physiological and pathophysiological significance are still not completely understood. The authors assert that the mechanoelectrical coupling is physiologically significant for regulation of functioning of normal myocardium, because it provides coordinated changes of the action potential and of the kinetics of intracellular calcium depending on the mechanical conditions, which is an additional contributing factor of the cardiac muscle adaptation to changing external conditions of mechanical contraction. The same authors acknowledge that arrhythmogenic effects of mechanical impacts are well-known; for example, a sharp shortening or quick mechanical stretches of cardiomyocytes under certain conditions lead to extra action potentials.

Moreover, after studying influence of myocardial heterogeneity on the efficiency of its mechanical function, the same authors come also to unexpected findings. It proved that "different types of mechanical heterogeneity (...) can play a positive or negative role depending on the distribution of heterogeneous properties and on the order the elements of the system are activated" [90]. In pathology, fine coordination of individual characteristics of cardiomyocytes and sequence of their activation can be broken, so that myocardial system becomes disorganized, and its function deteriorates. For example, parts with casual inclusions of hypoxic, hypertrophic and normal cardiomyocytes were observed in the mature myocardium, and therefore it happened that the functional properties of the cells in such a system (particularly, their electromechanical characteristics) were randomly distributed with respect to a sequence of excitation. As a result, the strength of cardiac contraction decreases sharply in such a system, while arrhythmogenic dispersion of repolarization increases. It has been shown that derangement of the accurate sequence of activation of the myocardium can lead to a sharp deterioration in its contractile function, and this fact helps to explain why so often the clinic use of artificial pacemaker does not improve the quality of life of patients. In that way, the complex and diversified investigation brought out clearly that cardiac arrhythmias can result not only from the disorder of the electrical activity of the heart, but also from disorder of its contractile function, and that the most important cause of arrhythmias is a disarrangement in the mechanisms of synchronous interaction between the electrical and mechanical processes in the myocardium.

Consequently, the term *"pathological cardiac arrhythmia" should be understood not only as these or those disorders in electrical activity of the heart, but it is disorders of its functioning as the whole organ*, which is a part of the entire cardiovascular system with its complex regulatory mechanisms.

If disorders in electrical organization of the heart are well compensated by the mechanical properties of multi-cellular system of the myocardium, the heart continues to perform its pump function effectively. On the contrary, very serious disorders of the pump function of the heart, caused by disorders in the accurate organization of the mechanical properties of the myocardial multi-cellular system, can occur even during the "normal" sequence of propagation of electric (i.e. autowave) excitation in the heart. Scientific observation of the heart from this new standpoint of biophysics and cybernetics makes us re-ask the question, in what cases changing the position of the source of excitation waves should be seen as a failure of adaptive mechanisms (i.e., as the disease), and in what cases such sorts of arrhythmia should still considered as a normal effect of adaptive mechanisms or as their side effect. In case of pathological arrhythmias, another task associated with revealing the exact location of failure of adaptation remains: whether it finds itself in the myocardium or in one of the control loops and guidance loops that serve the cardiac action.

Hence, according to the conception presented here, we must distinguish at least the following groups of pathological arrhythmias:

- arrhythmias that are ranked among normal reactions of adaptation, but, nevertheless, lead to hemodynamic disorders, dangerous for the whole organism (the mechanisms of regulation of population dynamics, for example);
- arrhythmias that result from disorders of adaptation because of disorganization in the chains of regulation of cardiac action;
- arrhythmias that result from disorders of adaptation because of disorganization of the autowave function of the heart.

It must be assumed that these new results will help finally to begin effective treatment of cardiac arrhythmias by restoring the accurate organization of such a complex system which the heart is indeed.

The biophysical language provides a better understanding of the causes of cardiac disorders, because it offers a number of integral characteristics of biological objects, and this is what gives him additional power. The physiological language has become actually a linguistic subset of the biophysical language, and it is quite a natural process in the development of knowledge.

Acknowledgements

Author is thankful for Dr. E. Shnol, Dr. Yu. Elkin, Prof. A. Loskutov, and Prof. A. Ardashev for interesting discussion of important aspects of modern cardiovascular physics. The partial support of Russian Foundation for Basic Research is acknowledged (the project 11-07-00519).

Author details

Andrey Moskalenko*

The Institute of Mathematical Problems of Biology, Russian Academy of Sciences, Pushchino, Russian Federation

References

[1] Moskalenko, A. Tachycardia as "Shadow Play". In: Takumi Yamada (ed.) Tachycardia. Rijeka: InTech; 2012; ISBN 978-953-51-0413-1. p97–122.

[2] Elkin, Yu. & Moskalenko, A. Basic mechanisms of cardiac arrhythmias. In: Ardashev A.V. (ed.) Clinical Arrhythmology. Moscow: MedPraktika-M; 2009; ISBN 978-5-98803-198-7. p45–74 (*in Russian*).

[3] Preliminary report: effect of encainide and flecainide on mortality in a randomized trial of arrhythmia suppression after myocardial infarction. The Cardiac Arrhythmia Suppression Trial (CAST) Investigators. New England Journal of Medicine 1989;321(6) 406–412. doi:10.1056/NEJM198908103210629.

[4] Brooks M.M., Gorkin L., Schron E.B., Wiklund I., Campion J., Ledingham R.B. Moricizine and quality of life in the Cardiac Arrhythmia Suppression Trial II (CAST II)". Controlled clinical trials 1994;15(6) 437–449.

[5] Golitsyn SP. Borders between benefits and risks in the treatment of ventricular disturbances of cardiac rhythm. International Journal of Medical Practice 2000;(10) 56–64.

[6] Druin Burch. Taking the Medicine: A Short History of Medicine's Beautiful Idea, and our Difficulty Swallowing It. London: Chatto & Windus (Random House); 2009. ISBN: 978-0701182786.

[7] Kurian, T. & Efimov I. Mechanisms of fibrillation: neurogenic or myogenic? Reentrant or focal? Multiple or single? Still puzzling after 160 years of inquiry. J Cardiovasc Electrophysiol. 2010;21(11) 1274–5, ISSN: 1540-8167.

[8] Mandel W. J., editor. Cardiac Arrhythmias: Their Mechanism, Diagnosis, and Management. Philadelphia, Pa: J.B. Lippincott; 1995; ISBN 978-039-75-1185-3.

[9] Schmidt R. F. and Thews G., editors. Human Physiology. Springer-Verlag, Berlin-Heidelberg-New York; 1983; ISBN: 3-540-11669-9.

[10] Sherwood L. Human Physiology: From Cells to Systems. Cengage Learning; 2013; ISBN: 9781133108931.

[11] Crampin EJ, Halstead M, Hunter P, Nielsen P, Noble D, Smith N & Tawhai M. Computational physiology and the physiome project. Experimental Physiology 2004;89(1) 1-26.

[12] Noble D. Modelling the heart — from Genes to Cells to the Whole Organ. Science 2002;295 1678-1682

[13] Noble D. Modelling the heart: Insights, failures and progress. BioEssays 2002;24 1156-1163.

[14] Wessel N, Malberg H, Bauernschmitt R & Kurths J. Nonlinear methods of cardiovascular physics and their clinic application. International Journal of Bifurcation and Chaos 2007;17(10) 3325-3371.

[15] Ewing GW. There is a need for an alternative or modified medical paradigm incorporating an understanding of the nature and significance of the physiological systems. North American Journal of Medical Science 2010;2(6) 246–251.

[16] Loskutov A. Fascination of chaos. Physics – Uspekhi 2010;53(12) 1257–1280.

[17] Loskutov A., Shavarov A.A., Dolgushina E.A., Ardashev A.V. Cardiac tissue as active media: Invariant characteristics of the theory of dynamical systems and heart rate variability. In: Ardashev A.V. (ed.) Clinical Arrhythmology. Moscow: MedPraktika-M; 2009, ISBN 978-5-98803-198-7. p1085–1103 (*in Russian*).

[18] Loskutov A. & Mironyuk O. Time series analysis of ECG: A possibility of the initial diagnostics. International Journal of Bifurcation and Chaos 2007;17(10) 3709-3713.

[19] Feigin, M. & Kagan, M. Emergencies as a manifestation of effect of bifurcation memory in controlled unstable systems. International Journal of Bifurcation and Chaos 2004;14(7) 2439–2447, ISSN 0218-1274.

[20] Ataullakhanov, F., Lobanova, E., Morozova, O., Shnol', E., Ermakova, E., Butylin, A. & Zaikin, A. Intricate regimes of propagation of an excitation and self-organization in the blood clotting model. Physics—Uspekhi 2007;50(1) 79–94, ISSN 1063-7869.

[21] Moskalenko, A. & Elkin, Yu. The lacet: a new type of the spiral wave behavior. Chaos, Solitons & Fractals, 2009;40(1) 426–431, ISSN 0960-0779

[22] Titomir LI. & Kneppo P. Bioelectric and Biomagnetic Fields. Theory and Applications in Electrocardiology. Boca. Ratón, Florida: CRC Press; 1994. ISBN 978-0849387005.

[23] Sahu P., Lim P.O., Rana B.S. and Struthers A.D. QT dispersion in medicine: electrophysiological Holy Grail or fool's gold? QJM: An International Journal of Medicine 2000;93(7) 425–431. DOI: 10.1093/qjmed/93.7.425.

[24] Baum O.V., Popov L.A., Voloshin V.I., Muromtseva G.A. QT-dispersion: Models and measurements. Bulletin of arrhythmology 2000;(20) 6–17 (*in Russian*). http://www.vestar.ru/atts/1669/166901.pdf

[25] Baum OV., Popov LA., Voloshin VI., Muromtseva GA. QT dispersion in orthogonal and pseudo-orthogonal lead systems. Bulletin of arrhythmology 2002;(26) 49–56 (*in Russian*). http://www.vestar.ru/atts/983/983baum.pdf

[26] Akintunde AA, Oyedeji AT, Familoni OB, Ayodele OE, Opadijo OG. QT Interval prolongation and dispersion: Epidemiology and clinical correlates in subjects with newly diagnosed systemic hypertension in Nigeria. J Cardiovasc Dis Res 2012;3(4) 290–295. DOI: 10.4103/0975-3583.102705.

[27] Trayanova N. Concepts of ventricular defibrillation. Phil. Trans. R. Soc. Lond. A 2001; (359) 1327–1337; DOI: 10.1098/rsta.2001.0834.

[28] Efimov IR, Cheng YN, Van Wagoner DR, Mazgalev, TN. & Tchou, P. J. Virtual electrode-induced phase singularity: a basic mechanism of defibrillation failure. Circ. Res. 1998;(88) 918–925.

[29] Efimov I.R., Kroll M.W., Tchou P.J., editors. Cardiac Bioelectric Therapy: Mechanisms and Practical Implications. Springer, 2008; ISBN 978-038-77-9403-7.

[30] Luther S, Fenton FH, Kornreich BG, Squires A, Bittihn P, Hornung D, Zabel M, Flanders J, Gladuli A, Campoy L, Cherry EM, Luther G, Hasenfuss G, Krinsky VI, Pumir A, Gilmour RF Jr, Bodenschatz E. Low-energy control of electrical turbulence in the heart. Nature 2011;475(7355):235-9. DOI: 10.1038/nature10216.

[31] Zhuchkova, E., Radnayev, B., Vysotsky, S. & Loskutov, A. Suppression of turbulent dynamics in models of cardiac tissue by weak local excitations. In: Dana S.K., Roy P.K., Kurths J. (eds.) Understanding Complex Systems. Berlin: Springer; 2009; p89–105.

[32] Winfree AT.Varieties of spiral wave behavior: An experimentalist's approach to the theory of excitable media. Chaos 1991;1(3) 303–334, ISSN 1054-1500

[33] Krinskii VI., Kokoz Iu.M. Analysis of the equations of excitable membranes. III. Purkinje fiber membrane. Reduction of the Noble equations to a 2d order system. Analysis of automaticity by nullcline graphs. Biofizika 1973;18(6) 1067-73.

[34] Moskalenko, A. Nonlinear effects of lidocaine on polymorphism of ventricular arrhythmias. Biophysics 2009;54(1) 47-50, ISSN 0006-3509.

[35] Starmer CF. How antiarrhythmic drugs increase the rate of sudden cardiac death. International Journal of Bifurcation and Chaos 2002;12(9) 1953-1968.

[36] Moskalenko, A. & Elkin, Yu. Is monomorphic tachycardia indeed monomorphic? Biophysics 2007;52(2) 237–240, ISSN 0006-3509.

[37] Prigogine I. From Being to Becoming: Time and Complexity in the Physical Sciences. San Francisco: W.H Freeman & Co; 1980. ISBN: 978-0716711079.

[38] Mikhailov A.S. Foundations of Synergetics. Berlin: Springer; 1990.

[39] Bushev M. Synergetics: Chaos, Order, Self-Organization. World Scientific Pub Co Inc.; 1994. ISBN: 978-9810212865.

[40] Wiener N.; Rosenblueth A. The mathematical formulation of the problem of conduction of impulses in a network of connected excitable elements, specifically in cardiac muscle. Arch. Inst. Cardiologia de Mexico 1946;16 (3–4) 205–265.

[41] Grekhova, M.T., editor. Autowave processes in systems with diffusion. Gorky: Institute of Applied Mathematics of the USSR Academy; 1981. (*in Russian*).

[42] Krinsky V.I., editor. Self-organization. Autowaves and structures far from equilibrium. Berlin: Springer; 1984.

[43] Mikhailov A.S. Distributed active systems. Berlin: Springer; 1992.

[44] Mikhailov A.S., Krinsky V.I. Rotating spiral waves in excitable media: the analytical results. Physica D 1983; 9: 346-371.

[45] Kopell N. and Howard L.N., Plane wave solutions to reaction diffusion equations. Studies in Appl. Math., 1973;52:291-328.

[46] Kopell N., Reaction-diffusion equations and pattern formation. In Studies in mathematical biology, S. Levin, ed. MAA Studies in Mathematics, Mathematical Association of America, 1978;15:191-205.

[47] Starmer CF. Initiation of excitation waves. Scholarpedia (2007);2(2) 1848, revision #129751. doi:10.4249/scholarpedia.1848

[48] Kechker M.I. Manual of Clinical Electrocardiology. Moscow; 2000. ISBN: 5-900518-24-9 (*in Russian*).

[49] Mazurov M.E. About the formation of the uniform rhythm in the sinoatrial node in the heart. Biofizika 2009;54(1) 81-88 (*in Russian*).

[50] Mazurov M.E. Control of the unified heart rhythm. Biofizika 2009;54(1) 89-96(*in Russian*).

[51] Pertsov A.M., Panfilov A.V., Medvedeva F.U. Instabilities of autowaves in excitable media associated with critical curvature phenomenon; Biofizika 1983;28 100-102.

[52] Rusakov AV, Panfilov AV, Medvinskii AB. Unidirectional block of propagation of a single autowave in a narrow gap and emergence of a two-dimensional reentry depends on geometry of the obstacle and on excitability of the media. Biofizika 2003;48(4) 722-726.

[53] Fast V.G., Kléber A.G. Role of wavefront curvature in propagation of cardiac impulse. Cardiovasc. Res. 1997;33(2): 258-271.

[54] Khramov R.N., Krinsky V.I. Stationary propagation velocities of the stable and unstable impulse. Dependence on membrane ionic currents. Biofizika 1977;22(3) 512. (*in Russian*).

[55] Khramov R.N. Circulation of an impulse in excitable medium. Critical size of the closed loop. Biofizika 1978;23(5) 871. (*in Russian*).

[56] Fife P.C. Singular perturbation and wave front techniques in reaction-diffusion problems. SIAM-AMS Proceedings 1976; 23-50.

[57] Aslanidi O.V. and Mornev O.A. Soliton-Like Regimes and Excitation Pulse Reflection (Echo) in Homogeneous Cardiac Purkinje Fibers: Results of Numerical Simulations. Journal of Biological Physics 1999;25(2-3) 149–164. DOI:10.1023/A:1005119218136

[58] Kozek J., Marek M. Wave reflection in reaction-diffusion equations. Phys.Rev.Lett. 1995;74(11) 2134-2137.

[59] Petrov V., Scott S. K., Shott S. K., Showalter K. Excitablity, wave reflection and wave spliting in a cubic autocatalysis reactio-diffusion system. Phil. Trans. R. Soc. A. 1994;347(1685) 631–642.

[60] Gaztañaga L., Marchlinskia F.E., Betenskya B.P. Mechanisms of cardiac arrhythmias. Rev Esp Cardiol. 2012;65(2) 174-85. DOI: 10.1016/j.rec.2011.09.020.

[61] Allessie M.A., Bonke F.I.M. Schopman F.J.G. Circus movement in rabbit atrial muscle as a mechanism of tachycardia. III. The "leading circle" concept: a new model of circus movement in cardiac tissue without the involvement of an anatomical obstacle. *Circ. Res.*, 1977; 41: 9.

[62] Zaikin A.N., Kawczynski A.L. Spatial effects in active chemical systems. Model of leading center. *J. Non. Equilib. Thermodyn.* 1977; 2 39

[63] Antzelevitch C., Jalife C., Moe G.K. Characteristics of reflection as a mechanism of reentrant arrhythmias and its relationship to parasystole. *Circulation* 1981;61 182–191.

[64] Lamanna V., Antzelevitch C., Moe G. Effect of lidocaine on conduction through depolarized canine false tendons and on a model of reflected reentry. *J. Pharm. Exp. Ther.* 1982 221 353–361.

[65] Rozanski G., Jafile J., Moe G. Reflected reentry in nonhomogeneous ventricular muscle as a mechanism of cardiac arrhythmias. Circulation 1984; 69 163-–173.

[66] Brugada P., Wellens H.J.J. The role of triggered activity in clinical ventricular arrhythmias. *Pace* 1984; 7: 260–271.

[67] Schechter E., Freeman C.C., Lazzara R. Afterdepolarization as a mechanism for the long QT syndrom. J. Am. Coll. Cardiol. 1984;3(6) 1556-61.

[68] Wit A.L., Rosen M.R. Afterdepolarizations and triggered activity. In: Fozzard H.A., Haber E., Jennings R.B., Kate A.M., Morgan H.E. (eds) The Heart and Circulatory System. New York: Raven Press, Publishers; 1986. p 1449-1490.

[69] Fozzard H.A. Afterdepolarizations and triggered activity. Basic Res. Cardiol. 1992; 87 Suppl 2 105-13.

[70] Kass R.S., Tsien R.W., Weingart R. Ionic basis of transient inward current induced by strophanthidin in cardiac Purkinje fibres. J. Physiol. 1978; 281, 209–226.

[71] Johnson N., Danilo P., Wit A.L., and Rosen M.R. Characteristics of initiation and termination of catecholamine-induced triggered activity in atrial fibers of the coronary sinus. Circulation 1986;74(5) 1168-1179.

[72] Rosen M.R., Gelband H., Merker C., Hoffman B.F. Mechanisms of digitalis toxicity. Effects of ouabain on phase four of canine Purkinje fiber transmembrane potentials. Circulation. 1973;47 681–689.

[73] Ferrier G.R., Saunders J.H., Mendez C. 1973. A cellular mechanism for the generation of ventricular arrhythmias by acetylstrophanthidin. Circ Res. 1973;32(5):600-609.

[74] Noble D. Ionic mechanisms determining the timing of ventricular repolarization: significance for cardiac arrhythmias. Annals of the New York Academy of Sciences 1992;644(1) 1–22.

[75] Hassard B.D., Kazarinoff N.D., Wan Y.-H. Theory and application of Hopf bifurcation. Cambridge: Cambridge University Press; 1981.

[76] Deco, G; Jirsa, VK Ongoing cortical activity at rest: criticality, multistability, and ghost attractors. J Neurosci 2012;32(10) 3366–75.

[77] Efimov I.R., Krinsky V.I., Jalife J. Dynamics of rotating vortices in the Beeler-Reuter model of cardiac tissue. Chaos, Solitons & Fractals 1995;5(3/4) 513-526.

[78] Keener J.P. The dynamics of 3-dimensional scroll waves in excitable media. Physica D 1988;31(2) 269-276.

[79] Biktashev V.N., Holden A.V., Zhang H. Tension of organizing filaments of scroll waves. Phyl. Trans. Roy. Soc. London, ser A 1994; 347: 611-630.

[80] Biktashev V.N., Holden A.V., Mironov S.F., Percov A.M., Zaitsev A.V. Three-dimensional organisation of re-entrant propagation during experimental ventricular fibrillation. Chaos, Solitons & Fractals 2002; 13(8): 1713-1733.

[81] Mantel R.-M., Barkley D. Parametric forcing of scroll-wave patterns in three-dimensional excitable media. Physica D 2001;149 107–122.

[82] Wiener N. Cybernetics or control and communication in the animal and the machine. New York — London; 1961.

[83] Fedorov V.F. Development of basic techniques of differential chronocardiography. PhD thesis (Dissertation for the degree of Candidate of Medical Sciences). Pirogov Russian State Medical University, Moscow; 2001. (*in Russian*).

[84] Anokhin PK. The essays on physiology of functional systems. Moscow: Medicine; 1975. (*in Russian*).

[85] Anokhin PK. Philosophical aspects of the theory of functional systems. Moscow: Nauka; 1978. (*in Russian*).

[86] Gasparyan S.A. etc. The concept of state health monitoring system of the Russian population. Approved by the Minister of Health, T.B. Dmitrieva and Chairman of the Presidential Committee on Information Policy, A.S. Golubkov. Moscow, 1996. (*in Russian*).

[87] Simonov PV. The emotional brain. Moscow: Nauka; 1981. (*in Russian*).

[88] Cherkashin AK, and Leshchenko Ya A. Mathematical Modeling and Quantitative Analysis of the Demographic and Ecological Aspects of Russian Supermortality. Mathematical Modelling of Natural Phenomena 2011;5(6) 243-258.

[89] Hauser MD. Moral Minds: How Nature Designed a Universal Sense of Right and Wrong. New York: HarperCollins; 2006.

[90] Katsnel'son L.B., Solov'eva O.E., Sul'man T.B., Konovalov P.V., Markhasin V.S. Simulation of mechanoelectrical coupling in cardiomyocytes under normal and abnormal conditions 2006;51(6) 917-926.

[91] Solovyova O.E. Markhasin V.S., Solovyova O., Katsnelson L.B., Protsenko Y., Kohl P., Noble D. Mechano-electric interactions in heterogeneous myocardium: development of fundamental experimental and theoretical models. Prog Biophys Mol Biol. 2003;82(1-3) 207-220.

[92] Kohl P. (Ed.), Sachs F. (Ed.), Franz MR. (Ed.). Cardiac Mechano-Electric Coupling and Arrhythmias. Publisher: OUP Oxford; 2011. ISBN: 978-0199570164

Chapter 2

Chronobiological Aspects of Impact of Apnoic Episode and Reoxygenation on the Electrical Myocardial Properties and Autonomic Nervous System Activity in Wistar Rats

Pavol Svorc, Ivana Bacova, Pavol Svorc, Jr.,
Monika Novakova and Alexander Marossy

Additional information is available at the end of the chapter

http://dx.doi.org/10.5772/57168

1. Introduction

The most commonly diagnosed sleep disordered breathing is obstructive (OSA) and central (CSA) sleep apnea. However, establishing the pathogenic mechanisms are not clear and precise contribution of OSA or CSA in the development of cardiovascular disease is not fully understood (Arias and Sanchez, 2007). Increased sympathetic activity induced by hypoxia, blood viscosity, inflammation (Chowdhuri et al., 2007; Patel and Rosen, 2007) or increased oxidative stress (Schulz et al., 2006) may mediate establishing pathogenesis. In both of these disorders are described serious complications significantly increasing the risk of arterial hypertension, coronary heart disease, heart rhythm disorders, including myocardial infarction. Similarly, CSA is accompanied by a variety of disorders of the heart, such as right ventricular dysfunction (afterload) (Bugress, 1998).

Apnea episodes produce not only short-term systemic hypoxia as well as hypercapnia and acidosis, where not only the myocardium is suffering disorders (Budhiraja and Quan, 2005; Schulz et al., 2006; Aronow, 2007; Patel and Rosen, 2007; Arias and Sanchez, 2007), but also the central nervous system. These clinical trials unambiguously ascribe the increased risk of cardiac events to apneic episodes occuring during sleep. In addition, respiratory alkalosis is also an extremely common and complicated problem affecting virtually every organ system in the body, the etiology of which may be related to pulmonary or extrapulmonary factors. However, not at all consider the effect of the recovery of oxygen delivery (reoxygenation) after

INTECH
open science | open minds

© 2014 Svorc et al.; licensee InTech. This is a paper distributed under the terms of the Creative Commons Attribution License (http://creativecommons.org/licenses/by/3.0), which permits unrestricted use, distribution, and reproduction in any medium, provided the original work is properly cited.

apneic episodes on the onset or development of ventricular arrhythmias. Reoxygenation after apneic episodes does not automatically normalize myocardial properties (electrophysiological and mechanical), but can also increase the risk of reoxygenation arrhythmias (Mubagwa et al., 1997; Shinmura et al., 1997). There are many cardiac effects of pulmonary hyperventilation-induced respiratory alkalosis including tachycardia, heart rhythm disorders (Foster et al., 2001) and supraventricular tachycardia caused by altered atrioventricular nodal conduction (Chen et al., 2001). Disorders of pulmonary ventilation are clearly considered to be proarrhythmogenic.

The timing of the transient risk state is dependent upon the synchronisation of the patient and not upon the time *per se*. After a transmeridian flight over several time zones, individuals will be out of phase for at least a short duration of time with their new surroundings. Information on the speed of the adjustment of the human circadian system is not available, but the system is probably in a transient state of internal desynchronisation for several days, depending on the magnitude of the longitudinal transmeridian displacement. It is commonly stated that it takes one day for every change in meridian. In shift workers, the degree of disturbance of circadian desynchronisation of physiological functions is in relation to its surroundings and may vary with the type of working hour shift. Also, the interaction of endogenous rhythms with environmental factors must be considered.

2. Chronobiology of the electrophysiological myocardial properties under apnoic episode and reoxygenation

It has been shown that all cardiac functions as well as the symptoms of cardiovascular diseases, including the various types of ventricular arrhythmias, morbidity and mortality, show circadian dependence (rhythmicity (Henry et al., 1990; Gilpin et al., 1990; Waterhouse et al., 2000). Knowledge regarding circadian variations of the electrophysiological myocardial properties of the heart and autonomic nervous system activity may help to more precisely evaluate the risk of ventricular arrhythmia incidence. The evidence in the literature regarding circadian patterns in arrhythmias is complicated by the fact that nearly all of the studies are confounded by a variety of factors independent of the intrinsic arrhythmogenic activity (Portaluppi and Hermida, 2007).

But, the circadian system is the foundation of the sleep-wake cycle, disorders and abnormalities in sleep are often connected with disorders or abnormalities in the circadian system. Circadian rhythm sleep disorders, such as jet lag syndrome (Auger and Morgenthaler, 2009) and shift work sleep disorder (Akerstedt and Wright, 2009), are those specifically attributed to dysfunctions or insufficiencies in the circadian system. Taking into consideration the preeminence of the circadian clock in timing sleep, it is likely that other sleep disorders are also linked to circadian system abnormalities (Richardson, 2005).

There are the clinical trials, which refer to fact that connection of the circadian rhythmicity of the cardiovascular events with apnoic episodes may have practical relevance in screening for patients with OSA and may have prognostic clinical value in predicting future cardiovascular

events. The risk of sudden death from cardiac causes has peak from 06:00h to noon and a nadir from midnight to 06:00h. OSA is associated with neurohormonal and electrophysiological abnormalities that may increase the risk of sudden death from cardiac causes, especially during sleep. Gami et al. (2005) followed this dependence in 112 people, who died suddenly from cardiac causes. They found that from midnight to 06:00h, sudden death from cardiac causes occurred in 46% of people with OSA, as compared with 21% of people without OSA. People with sudden death from cardiac causes from midnight to 06:00h had a significantly higher apnea-hypopnea index than those with sudden death from cardiac causes during other intervals, and the apnea-hyponea index correlated directly with the relative risk of sudden death from cardiac causes from midnight to 06:00h. Thus, people with OSA have a peak in sudden death from cardiac causes during the sleeping hours, which contrasts strikingly with the nadir of sudden death from cardiac causes during this period in people without OSA. The different variation in onset of myocardial infarction was found in patients with and without OSA. Myocardial infarction occurred between 12:00h and 06:00h in 32% of OSA patients and 7% of non/OSA patients. Of all patients having myocardial infarction between 12:00h and 06:00h, 91% had OSA. These findings suggest that OSA may be a trigger for myocardial infarction and patients having nocturnal onset of myoacardial infarction should be evaluated for OSA. Future research should address the effects of OSA therapy for prevention of nocturnal cardiac events (Kuniyoshi et al., 2008).
Besides humans, almost all animals are exposed to periodic repetitions of light and dark cycles during a 24-hour (circadian) period to which virtually all physiological functions are synchronized. Disturbance of the internal synchronization of rhythms with the periodicity of the external environment may manifest by increased susceptibility to disease. Surprisingly, there are only few works describing day-time of the experiment running or synchronization of animals to the external environmental periodicity, such as the light-dark (LD) cycle. It can be a problem, because the LD cycle is given for one of the strongest circadian synchronizators of the animal endogenous rhythms. Therefore, the creation of experimental, *in vivo,* chronobiological animal models may help reveal some of the relationships between circadian time and biological function, which is sometimes very difficult to study in humans. From this reason, the circadian variability should be considered as important factor especially in the cardiovascular studies.

For example, the 24h course of the myocardial vulnerability showed the highest susceptibility of the rat ventricular myocardium to arrhythmias between 12:00h and 15:00h and highest resistance between 24:00h and 03:00h under normooxic conditions (Svorc et al., 1994; 2012). In hypoventilatory rat model, hypoventilation-induced systemic hypoxia, hypercapnia and acidosis increased the myocardial vulnerability and decreased heart rate values throughout the 24-hour period. Circadian rhythm of the electrical stability of the heart was changed to biphasic with smaller peak between 15:00h and 18:00h and higher peak between 24:00h and 03:00h. The hypoventilatory circadian rhythm of the electrical stability of the heart was not significant as revealed by the population mean cosinor (Svorc et al., 1997, 2000). Hyperventilation does not disturb, but likely only modifies the circadian rhythm of the electrical stability of the heart. The hyperventilatory 24h rhythm of the myocardial vulnerability shows a nonsignificant pattern, with higher myocardial resistance during the dark (active) period of the LD cycle.

On the basis of these facts, it is clear that the disorders of pulmonary ventilation (hypoventilation, hyperventilation) not only change the electrophysiological properties of the myocardium, but also circadian rhythm of the myocardial vulnerability to the ventricular arhythmias. This includes also apnoic episodes, which are also arrhythmogenicly. Problems of connection of the circadian rhythmicity of the cardiovascular system with apnoic episodes is not study in more detail, although clinical studies suggest a connection between sudden death from cardiac causes and OSA dependent on circadian timing. The question remains whether there also a reverse connection? Could patients with OSA, without obvious cardiac diseases, be more susceptible to heart-rhythm disorders during sleep after a change in synchronisation with local time? We evaluated if apneic episodes and subsequent reoxygenation changed the electrical predisposition of the heart to ventricular arrhythmias, heart rate (HR), activity of the autonomic nervous system and acid–base balance by the same manner in active (dark) and non-active (light) part of the day.

The present study conformed with the Guide for the Care and Use of Laboratory Animals published by the US National Institutes of Health (NIH publication number 85-23, revised 1996). The study protocol was also approved by the Ethics Committee of the Medical Faculty of Safarik University (Kosice, Slovak Republic) (permission number 2/05).

The experiments were performed in ketamine/xylazine anaesthetized female Wistar rats (ketamine [Narkamon] 100 mg/kg [SPOFA Prague] + xylazine [Rometar] 15 mg/kg, intramuscularly). Anaesthesia was maintained at a level such that painful stimuli and surgery did not evoke noticeable motor or cardiovascular responses. On completion of the experiments, rats were sacrificed by cardiac administration of an overdose of ketamine. The effect of the light period (light phase) on electrophysiological properties of the heart, acid-base balance, ions and heart rate variability (HRV) were followed after adaptation to an LD cycle (12h light, 12h dark, 40%-60% humidity, room temperature 24 °C, two animals/cage with access to food and water *ad libitum*) for four weeks, with the dark part of the cycle from 18:00h to 06:00h. The effect of the dark period (dark phase) was followed after adaptation to the inverse setting of the LD cycle (12h dark, 12h light), with the dark period from 06:00h to 18:00h. The experiments were performed twice (the first animal between 09:00h and 10:00h and the second animal between 12:00h and 13:00h) (scheme 1).

2.1. Ventilation

The trachea was exposed at the mid-cervical level and cannulated using a plastic tube. A tracheal cannula was attached to a volume-rate-regulated artificial ventilator (UGO Basile, Comerio-Varese, Italy) and animals ventilated by room air. The parameters of the initial ventilation and reoxygenation were a respiratory rate of 50 breaths/min and a tidal volume of 1 ml/100 g body weight. The parameters of ventilation were chosen on the basis of validated methods of artificial controlled ventilation using room air for pentobarbital-anaesthetised rats, which can be applied for the preservation of normal acid–base balance. Apneic episode was simulated by switching off the ventilator for 2 min. The respiratory effect of the pulmonary

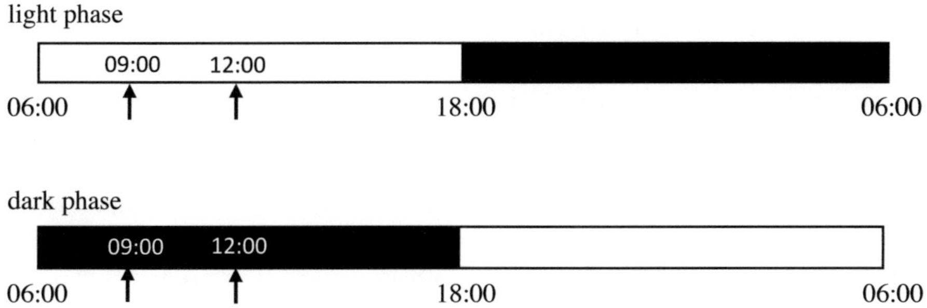

Scheme 1. Adaptation of rats to the LD cycle (12h : 12h) in a special room. Light stripe - the light part of the rat regime day, dark stripe - the dark part of the rat regime day. Arrows indicate the time of the experiment running.

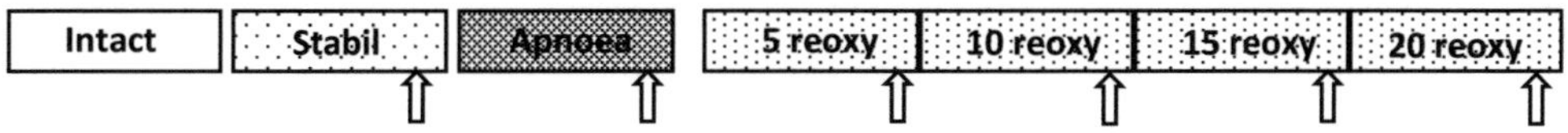

Scheme 2. Experimental protocol. Arrows denote single steps of the experiment with measurement of the ventricular arrhythmia threshold for evaluation of the electrical stability of the heart.

ventilatory changes was monitored by the analysis of the acid-base balance from blood samples taken from the femoral artery unrepeatedly at the end of experiment in the single groups.

2.2. Experimental protocol

Animals were randomly divided into seven groups (14 animals in each group) for the light and dark parts of the day to evaluate the acid–base balance in single experimental steps. Group 1 contained intact rats before surgical interventions, spontaneous breathing under ketamine/ xylazine anaesthesia (Intact). Group 2 contained rats after tracheotomy, thoracotomy and 5 min of normal artificial ventilation (Stabil). Group 3 contained rats who underwent 2 min of apnoea (Apnoea). Group 4 had rats that underwent 5 min of reoxygenation (5 reoxy). Group 5 had rats that underwent 10 min of reoxygenation (10 reoxy). Group 6 involved rats who had 15 min of reoxygenation (15 reoxy). Group 7 contained animals that had 20 min of reoxygenation (20 reoxy) after 2 min. apneic episode. The experiment was completed by taking blood samples (scheme 2).

2.3. Measurements

ECG parameters, acid-base balance and HRV measurements were performed in the supine position on a preheated table. Body temperature was maintained at a level equivalent to the rectal temperature measured before anaesthetic agent administration. Heat provided by an infrared lamp was used to prevent any hypothermic effects on heart rate.

The chest was opened via a parasternal thoracotomy for elimination of nervous breathing control mechanisms and measurement of the electrical stability of the heart (measured by the ventricular arrhythmia threshold - VAT). The VAT was estimated as the minimal amount of electrical current (mA) needed for elicitation of ventricular arrhythmias. The heart was protected from changes in temperature and humidity by administering physiological solution, dropwise, to the heart, with temperature equal to rectal temperature measured before the anaesthetic agent application. The stimulating platinum electrodes (diameter 1 mm and 5 mm interelectrode distance, temperatura equal to rectal temperature) were placed at the base of right ventricle. Parameters of the electrical stimulation were 400 ms series of rectangular pulses; frequency, 30 Hz; impulse length, 10 ms). Stimuli were triggered by onset of the R wave in the II lead of electrocardiography (ECG) on the base of synchronization of ECG with stimulator. The current intensity was increased progressively by increments of 0.2 mA until ventricular arrhythmias were obtained. Recovery of the sinus rhythm was spontaneous.

The bipolar electrodes were attached to the upper and lower limbs and served for recording of the heart rate (HR), ECG and heart rate variability (HRV). ECG was further analysed using computer software (ECG Practic Veterinary, Prague, Czech Republic). Measurement of the ECG and HR (mean value of the last four cycles) were carried out: in intact animals; after tracheotomy (Tr); thoracotomy (To); after each minute of the 5-min stabilization; after each 30 s of the apneic episode; and after each minute of the 20-min reoxygenation. HRV was analysed from ECG using computer software (Varia Pulse TF4, Sima, Olomouc, Czech Republic). Analysis of HRV was performed by scoring 600 RR intervals needed for calculation of HRV parameters. The following HRV parameters were measured: RR interval duration (ms), very low frequency (VLF) power (corresponding to sympathetic activity), low frequency (LF) power (baroreceptor activity, or sympathetic and parasympathetic activity together), high-frequency (HF) power (corresponding to parasympathetic activity) (ms^2) and relative VLF power, relative LF power and relative HF power (%).

2.4. Statistical analysis

The data are presented as the means ± SD. A non-paired t - test was used for statistical evaluation. Differences of $p < 0,05$ were considered significant. The relationship between the evaluated parameters was determined by calculating correlation coefficients. The interval $-0,4 > r > +0,4$ was considered to be significant. The data were processed from trials that were conducted independent of the season because circannual variation can also occur in the parameters that were examined.

2.5. Limitations of study

Absence of the reference ECG values, acid-base balance parameters and HRV parameters (also literary current data) from animals without anaesthesia and in the LD dependence can be a limitation in our study. The next limitation can be a relatively large dispersion of the measured values. The ECG, acid-base and HRV values showed intra- and interindividual variability, which is a problem, mainly concerning *in vivo* studies. The discrepancy can be explained by the production of spontaneous, unpredictible alterations in the electrophysiologic properties of the heart induced by anaesthesia, or hormonal and homeostatic reflexes in the animals. The third limitation was that rats were in systemic asphyxia from the start to the end of the experiment independent of the LD cycle. This state has been described by other authors in rats

(Sumitra et al., 2004; Alva et al., 2006) and reflects the changes in cardiovascular (Sumitra et al., 2004) and respiratory (Farver et al., 1986) systems.

In the first moment, we have focused on the assessment of the changes in heart rate and electrical stability of the heart. The disruptive effect of acute hypoxia on the LD-dependent differences in the HR–response curve was not confirmed, as suggested by other authors (Mortola and Seifert, 2000; Bishop et al., 2001; Bosco et al., 2003; Kaplan et al., 2003; Mortola, 2007). However, it is known that ketamine/xylazine anaesthesia decreases heart rate (Hsu et al., 1986; Morita et al., 1997; Cope et al., 1997) which has been connected with systemic asphyxia after administration of anaesthetic agent (Švorc et al., 2009).

One of the main conclusions is that the HR was significantly and systematically higher in the dark part than in the light part of the day during apneic episode-induced acute systemic asphyxia. Start of apneic episode significantly (p<0,001) decreased the HR only in the dark part of the day compared with the HR value from the end of the period of stabilization, not in the light part. The HR decreased gradually until the end of the apneic episode in both lighted parts of the day. Although reoxygenation significantly (p<0,001) increased the HR in both lighted parts of the day, surprising was the finding that the LD differences were eliminated during reoxygenation.

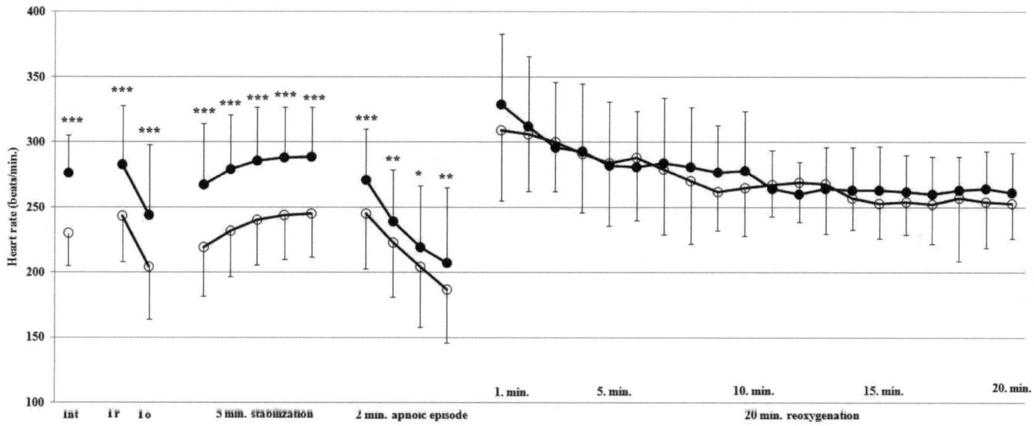

Figure 1. HR changes in single experimental steps. White circles represent the light part of the day and black circles the dark part. Int: intact animals under ketamine/xylazine anaesthesia before surgical intervention allowing for spontaneous breathing in the supine position. Tr: tracheotomy. To: thoracotomy.*** p < 0,001; ** p < 0,01 * p < 0,05 statistically significant HR differences between the light and dark part of the day (Svorc Jr. et al., 2011).

Twenty minutes of reoxygenation recovered the HR approximately to the HR levels of spontaneously breathing animals. Decrease of HR can be explained by effect of hypoxia (Hinojosa-Laborde and Mifflin, 2005) or a larger parasympathetic influence (Hayashida et al., 1996; Svorc Jr. et al. 2013) (figure 1).

The electrical stability of the heart after the period of stabilization showed significant (p<0,001) LD differences with the higher values during the active (dark) part of the regimen day. Apneic episodes significantly (p<0,001) decreased the VAT in both light parts of the day and eliminated LD differences. The results clearly demonstrate and confirm the pro-arrhythmogenic effects of apneic episodes (Budhiraja and Quan, 2005; Schulz et al., 2006; Aronow, 2007; Patel and Rosen, 2007; Arias and Sanchez, 2007). In our model, we initially stated that the pro-arrhythmogenic effects of apneic episodes act in the same manner regardless of whether they are in the light (non-active) or dark (active) part of the day for rats (figure 2).

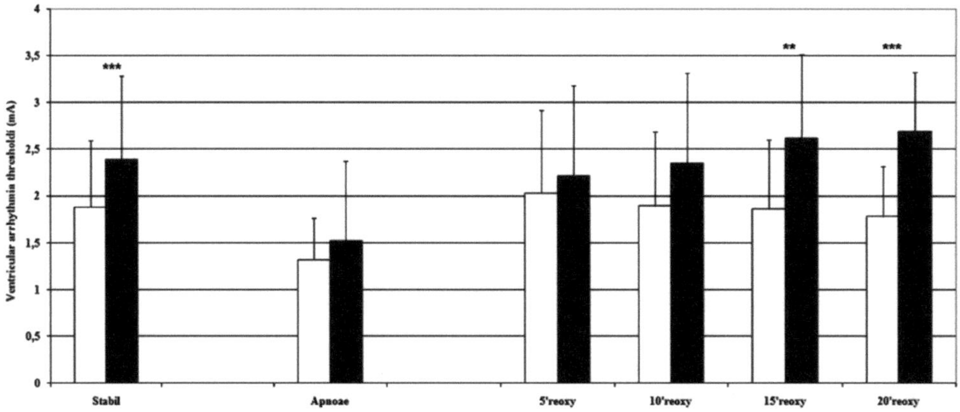

Figure 2. VAT changes in single experimental steps. White columns represent the light part of the day, and black columns the dark part. Stabil: animals after tracheotomy, toracotomy and 5 min artificial ventilation. Apnoae: after a 2-min apneic episode. 5 reoxy, 10 reoxy, 15 reoxy and 20 reoxy: after 5, 10, 15 and 20 min of reoxygenation, respectively. *** p < 0,001; ** p < 0,01 statistically significant VAT differences between the light and dark part of the day (Svorc Jr. et al., 2011).

The decreased the electrical stability of the heart also in the course of whole 24h period (Svorc et al., 1994, 1997) confirm results from other electrophysiological studies about the effect of hypoxia on myocardium. The reason of disorders of the heart rhythm in the hypoxic state is a sudden increase of the extracellular K^+ concentration, which play the crucial role in the changes of the rest membrane potential and can produce the ectopic activity as well as inhibition of the rapid reaction (Opie et al., 1979). The rapid increase of the extracellular K^+ concentration is result of K_{ATP} channel activation. It is inactivated in the normooxic conditions, but it is activated in the hypoxic or anoxic conditions (Noma and Shibasaki, 1985; Sanguinetti et al., 1988; Daut et al., 1990; Billman et al., 1993). Thus, the blockade of K_{ATP} channels acts antiarrhythmic (Wolleben et al., 1989). We can suppose that mechanism of the K^+ current activation by hypoxia can be responsible for change in the electrical stability of the heart also in the circadian dependence, although biphasic course of the VAT is not perspicuously explained by this mechanism.

However, it seems that recovery of the pulmonary ventilation after apneic episodes can also contribute to heart rhythm disorders, but this is dependent upon the light (non-active)-dark (active) cycle. In the dark part of the day, the gradual increase in the VAT is associated with the duration of reoxygenation (anti-arrhythmogenic effect) compared with the light part of the day, where the contrary tendency was observed (pro-arrhythmogenic effect). This suggests that synchronisation of the organism to a particular enviromental periodicity could be a crucial factor influencing myocardial vulnerability to ventricular arrhythmias mainly in the process of recovery of the pulmonary ventilation after an apneic episode. Our model suggests that synchronisation to local time may be an important factor for evaluation of cardiovascular risk in patients suffering from OSA. Analyses of myocardial reactions to acute systemic asphyxia induced by apneic episodes (as well as to reoxygenation) is very important in experimental respirology and cardiology because the myocardium reacts differently depending on the external environmental periodicity.

3. Chronobiology of the ECG parameters during apnoic episode and reoxygenation

Therefore, myocardial vulnerability changes depend on the breathing as well as on the lighted mode of the rat regime day. In addition, number of electrophysiological properties of the cardiac structures are recognized as essential for the triggering and maintenance of heart rhythm disorders and show dependence on the time of day (Portaluppi and Hermida, 2007). The question remains, which electrophysiological properties play a role in the myocardial sensitivity to the ventricular arrhythmias during apnoic episode and recovery of the pulmonary ventilation (reoxygenation) depending on the cycle of the light and the darkness succession. Ventilatory disorders act arrhythmogenicly and the chronophysiological view on the functional interconnection between disorders of pulmonary ventilation and changes in the electrophysiologic properties of the heart are also important. We got from the fact that ventricular arrhythmias may arise either from the disorders of the impulse formation and conduction (presented by PQ interval), or from a enlarged dispersion of the refractory periods (presented by QT interval).

We analyzed the PQ and QT interval changes (Bacova et al., 2010) in the single experimental steps. In intact animals, higher values of PQ interval duration during in the light (inactive, sleep) phase of the rat regime day suggest that ventricular myocardium is more susceptible to arrhythmias originating from impulse production and conduction compare to the active part of the day. The speed of the impulse conduction from atria to ventricles (PQ interval) depends from action potential amplitude, reflecting the active role of Na^+ channels (Carmeliet, 1986; Amitzur et al., 2000). It can mean that ketamine/xylazine anaesthesia with associated systemic asphyxia as well as with subsequent surgical interventions do not affect the kinetics of the Na $^+$ channels, which are likely to be different in the light and dark part of the rat regime day. It seems that PQ interval is the relative stable electrophysiological parameter of the heart and it is directly influenced by the LD cycle (figure 3). Mechanisms of such different effect of ketamine/xylazine anaesthesia are still unknown and were not analyzed in detail.

Apneic episodes, obstructive or central, often in a connection with the sleep apnea syndrome, are linked with disorders of the cardiac rhythm (Cutler et. al., 2002; Yamashita et al., 2004; Bounhoure et al., 2005; Dunai et al., 2006; Bayram and Diker, 2008; Grešová et al., 2009). In our

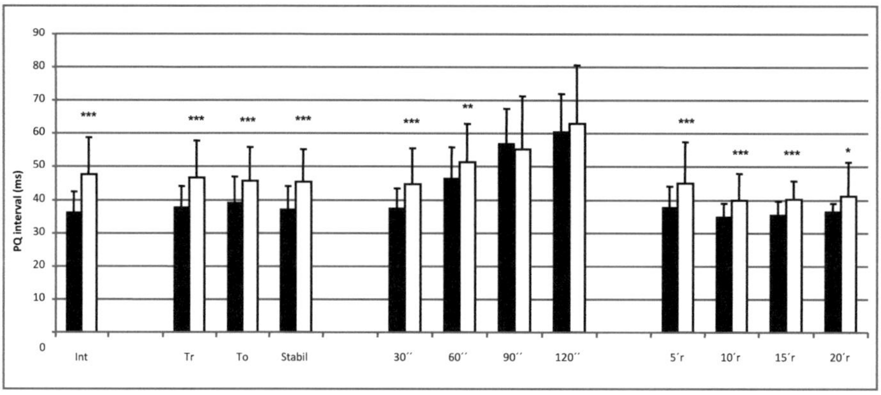

Figure 3. Mean ± SD values of the PQ interval duration in intact animals (Int), after tracheotomy (Tr), thoracotomy (To), 5 min. stabilization (Stabil), in each 30 sec. of 2 minutes apneic episode and after 5., 10., 15. and 20 minute of artificial reoxygenation.. Empty and black columns refer to light and dark parts of the day, respectively. The level of significance of differences between the light and dark part of the rat regime day is indicated by the symbol (* p < 0,05, ** p < 0,01, *** p < 0,001) (Bacova et al., 2010).

model, short-term asphyxia increases vulnerability to the arrhythmias originating from disorders of the impulse production and conduction more in the light (inactive) than in the dark (active) part but does not disturb LD dependence. Long-term apneic episode, connected with more serious asphyxia, henceforth prolonges PQ interval and increases vulnerability to the arrhythmias but probably independently on the LD cycle. Reoxygenation recovered PQ interval duration to the pre-asphyxic values with preservation of the LD differences observed in intact animals.

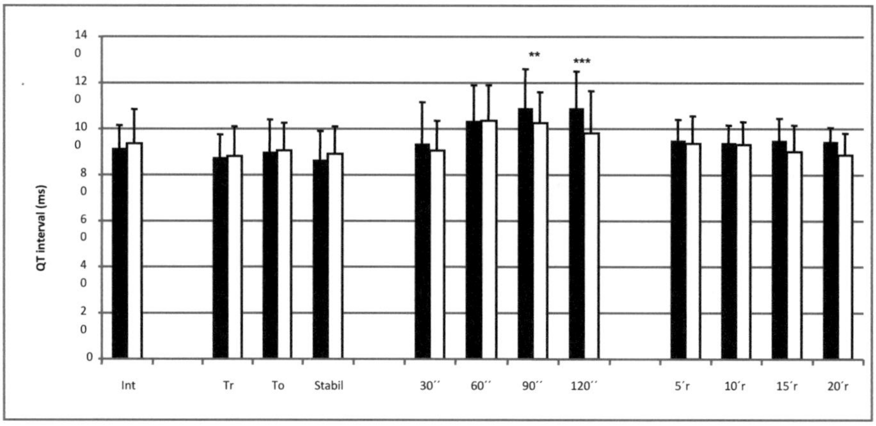

Figure 4. Mean ± SD values of the QT interval duration in intact animals (Int), after tracheotomy (Tr), thoracotomy (To), 5 min. stabilization (Stabil), in each 30 sec. of 2 minutes apneic episode and after 5., 10., 15. and 20 minute of artificial reoxygenation. Empty and black columns refer to light and dark parts of the day, respectively. The level of significance of differences between the light and dark part of the rat regime day is indicated by the symbol (* p < 0,05, ** p < 0,01, *** p < 0,001) (Bacova et al., 2010).

Loss of the LD differences in the dispersion of the refractory period durations (QT interval) can be a result of the effect of the initial asphyxia, which has distracting influence on the LD differences in QT interval. A similar situation was described by Gunes et al. (2008) in clinical study, where the loss of diurnal variation of the dispersion of the refractory periods was also present in patients having either an ischemic or non-ischemic origin of heart failure treated with optimal drug therapy. Although dispersion of the refractory period duration (QT interval) is the result of the action of more ion currents (Ca^{2+}, Na^{+}, Cl^{-} and inward rectifying K^{+} current) (Amitzur et al., 2000), depends mainly from intracellular K^{+} concentration (Froldi et al., 1994). This suggests that ketamine/xylazine anaesthesia together with initial asphyxia probably influence mainly K^{+} ion current by the same manner in the both lighted parts of the day and disturb the light-dark dependence.

The opposite situation is true of the QT interval. Short-term apneic episode increased vulnerability to the arrhythmias originating from dispersion of the refractory period independently on the LD cycle, but long-term apneic episode facilitated the LD differences with the higher dispersion during the dark (active) than light (nonactive) part of the rat daily regime. The next LD difference was seen at the end of asphyxic period. Slightly decreased the QT interval duration was only during the light (nonactive) part, but not during the dark (active) one.

These changes may be caused by changes in ion channel sensitivities regarding duration and gravity of asphyxia. Hypoxia exacerbated the atrioventricular conduction by reduction of the slow inward Na^{+} current and by rectifying K^{+} current and depressed automaticity by the increase of the outward K^{+} current and in the certain range by reduction of the slow inward Na^{+} current in the isolated rabbit AV node (Nishimuraet al., 1989). Sinus interval, AH and HV interval are gradually prolonged with the duration of the hypoxia. These effects are attributed to the $K^{+}{}_{ATP}$ channel (Sawanobori 1995), which is probably activated by the endogenous adenosine released from the hypoxic myocardium (Xu et al., 1994; Leone Jr. and Merrill, 1995). Our results suggest that above mentioned changes can be modified also by the LD cycle.

Interesting is fact that the average values of QT interval were slightly and nonsignicantly longer in the dark part of the day after reoxygenation compared to the light one, while the opposite tendency was observed in the intact animals and after stabilization. These slight differences probably do not have any biological significance because they may be a result of the relatively large variation in dispersion of the refractory periods, what corresponds with second limitation (Lubbe et al., 1975). Similarly, there are contrary conclusions about the effect of reoxygenation on the changes of the electrophysiological myocardial properties. Our results affirm the opinion of some authors about the antiarrhythmogenic effect of reoxygenation (Perchenet and Kreher, 1995; Bugge et al., 1997). There are papers however, which describe the serious injury of the heart by the reoxygenation (Griffiths et al., 2000; Mukai et al., 2000).

What is known about the effects of hypoxia on circadian patterns is still quite limited, especially with respect to the causative mechanistic sequence of the hypoxic effects. It appears that the most common effect of prolonged hypoxia is to decrease, and in come cases to abolish, the amplitudes of the daily oscillations, irrespective of the state of arousal or activity level. On the other hand, the evidence is that hypoxia causes only minimal and transient perturbation of the period of the rhythm. The fact that hypoxia modifies the circadian oscillations of variables as important as body temperature and metabolism leads to the expectation that the daily rhythms of many other functions are perturbed by hypoxia, according to their link to the primary variables (Mortola, 2007). This modification can be probably seen also in our experimental model, where the definite loss of the LD dependence was not demonstrated in followed parameters of ECG.

4. Chronobiology and autonomic nervous system during apnoic episode and reoxygenation

Circadian rhythms in autonomic nervous system activity are well known that directly controls circadian thythm in cardiovascular system and constitute major triggers of cardiac arrhythmias. Increased sympathetic activity accelerates heart rate, favors spontaneous depolarization, shortens the ventricular effective refractory period, and decrease the threshold for ventricular fibrillation. In contrast, increased parasympathetic activity slows heart rate, decreases AV nodal conduction, and in the presence of baseline sympathetic neural activity, increases both the ventricular refractory period and the ventricular fibrillation threshold (review of references in Portaluppi and Hermida, 2007). This direct and clear dependence, described in people and in larger experimental animals, was not confirmed in rats (Svorc et al., 1994, 1997).

OSA is associated with increased daytime and nocturnal sympathetic activity, what can be the risk factor of cardiovascular disease. It is associated with a significant worsening in heart-rate variability, heart rate turbulence and QT dynamicity parameters (Aytemir et al., 2007). Its mechanism can be explained by the observation that the sympathetic tone increases due to repetitive apneas accompanied by hypoxias and arousals during sleep. Heart rate variability representing cardiac autonomic function is mediated by respiratory sinus arrhythmia, baroreflex-related fluctuation and thermoregulation-related fluctuation. The LF/HF ratio was higher in the severe OSA syndrome group to that of the moderate group (Park et al., 2008). Structural changes occur in the airway to obstruct airflow during OSA, and the resulting apnea activates hypoxic and hypercapnic reflexes, wich in turn lead to profound elevation in sympathetic nerve activity and cyclical changes in parasympathetic nerve activity. These autonomic effects are though to contribute to the associated cardiovascular diseases (eg, hypertension) and frequently observed brady- and tachyarrhythmias (Cutler et al., 2002). Autonomic abnormalities seen in pacient with OSA include increased resting heart rate, decreased RR interval variability and increased blood pressure variability (Parish and Somers, 2004). Using heart rate variability analysis, nocturnal sinusal dysfunction contrasted with a blunted diurnal parasymathetic modulation of the sinus node. Frequent nocturnal nonsustained supraventricular tachycardias were predominantly found in patients with severe sleep related breathing disorders; however, an increased risk of ventricular arrhythmias was not found. (Roche et al., 2003).

Apneic episodes influence the autonomic nervous system activity (Aydin et al., 2004), but little is know about the effect on circadian variation in this system activities. The circadian rhythm of the LF, HF and LF/HF ratio differed significantly in the group of patients with mild OSA (group 2, apnea index AI > or = 20) compared with group of patients with severe OSA (group 1, apnea index AI < 20) and control group. The mean HF from 04:00h to 12:00h was significantly lower in group2 than in group1 and the control group, and it correlated significantly with the lowest nocturnal O_2 saturation (r = 0,58). The mean LF/HF ratio during the same period was significantly higher in group2 than in group1 and the control group, and it correlated significantly with total time of the nocturnal oxygen saturation < 90% (r = 0,64) and the lowest nocturnal O_2 saturation (r = 0,56). These findings suggest that sleep-disordered breathing associated with severe oxygen desaturation might influence heart rate variability not only sleep but also during daytime. OSA per se might contribute to altered circadian rhythm in autonomic activity leading to the development of cardiovascular diseases (Noda et al., 1998) also in the absence of hypertension, heart failure, or other disease states, and that it is linked to the severity of OSA (Aydin et al., 2004). These conclusions were supported by Tükek et al. (2003) in study, where examined the possible effect of diurnal variability of heart rate on the development of arrhythmias in patients with chronic obstructive pulmonary disease. They concluded that patients with chronic obstructive pulmonary disease with arrhythmia had circadian disturbances in heart rate variability such as unchanged night-time parasympathetic tone and disturbed sympathovagal balance in favour of the sympathetic system all day long, which may explain the increased frequency of arrhythmia.

The next step in the analysis of the effect of apnoic episode and reoxygenation on the electrical stability of the heart was assessment of the changes in the activity of the autonomic nervous system in LD dependence. The HRV was applied to assess these changes. HRV was not evaluated during apnoic episode because the changes in the duration of the RR intervals drastically have been extended, resulting in a high dispersion of the values.

The first 5 minutes of recovery pulmonary ventilation has been associated with significant turbulence in the heart rhythm, especially in the light part of the day (time range of R-R interval ranged from 0.025 to ms 0,717 ms). In a dark part of the day, so a significant dispersion was not observed. Although the LD differences were not maintained during the 20-minute reoxygenation, in the light part has been observed nonsignificant the tendency of the shortening compare to the dark part, where the duration of the RR interval was prolonged. These results coincide with heart rate changes. Reoxygenation recovered RR interval duration to the values from intact animals only in the dark (active) part (figure 5).

Significant LD differences in power HF were seen in the intact animals with the higher value in the light part compared to the dark one. Effect of reoxygenation on the power HF has been dependent on the LD cycle. Power HF gradually increased and reached a level of intact animals with the time of the reoxygenation but only in the dark part of the rat regime day. In the light part of the day, the changes in the power HF were nesignificant and fluctuated randomly, without any tendency of decrease or increase. Significant LD differences were maintained throughout the period of reoxygenation, up to the 20th minute, where the elimination of this difference has been observed. In each interval evaluation of power HF, the value was higher in the dark compare to light part of the day (figure 6). Reoxygenation did not recover power HF, but preserved the dominant position of the parasympathetic division in the both lighted periods.

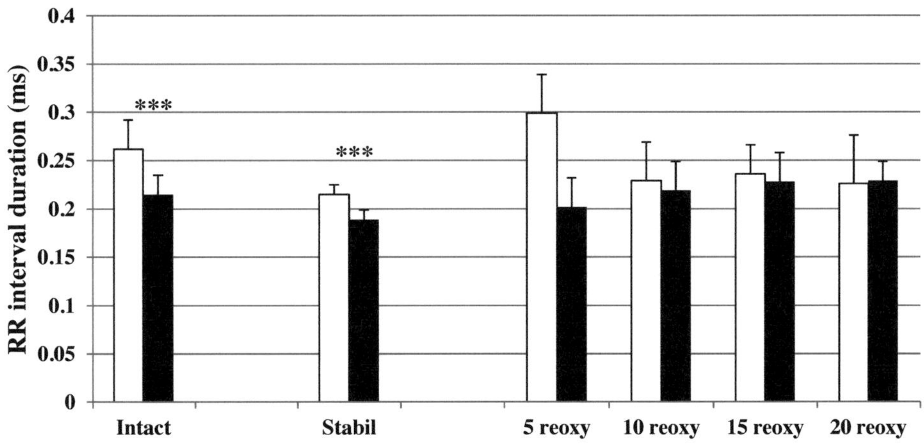

Figure 5. Mean ± SD values of the RR interval duration in intact animals (Intact), after tracheotomy, thoracotomy and 5 min. stabilization (Stabil) and after 20 minute of artificial reoxygenation. Empty and black columns refer to light and dark parts of the day, respectively. The level of significance of differences between the light and dark part of the rat regime day is indicated by the symbol (*** p < 0,001).

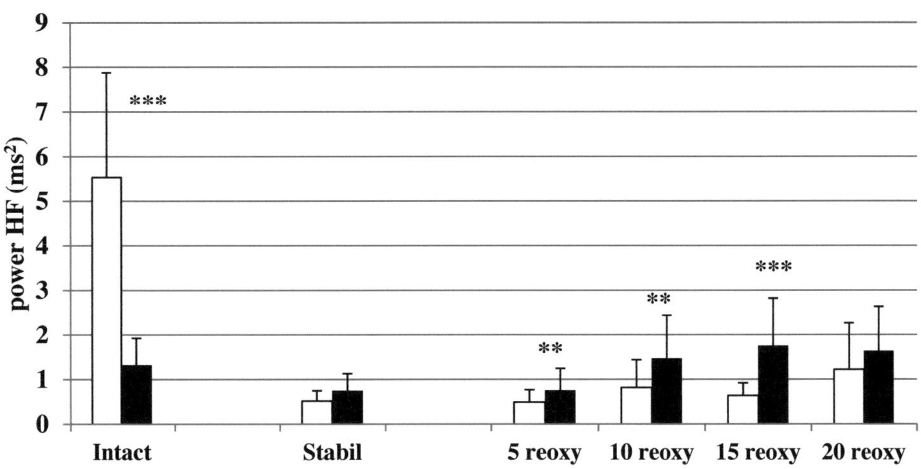

Figure 6. Mean ± SD values of the power HF in intact animals (Intact), after tracheotomy, thoracotomy and 5 min. stabilization (Stabil) and after 20 minute of artificial reoxygenation. Empty and black columns refer to light and dark parts of the day, respectively. The level of significance of differences between the light and dark part of the rat regime day is indicated by the symbol (** p < 0,01, *** p < 0,001).

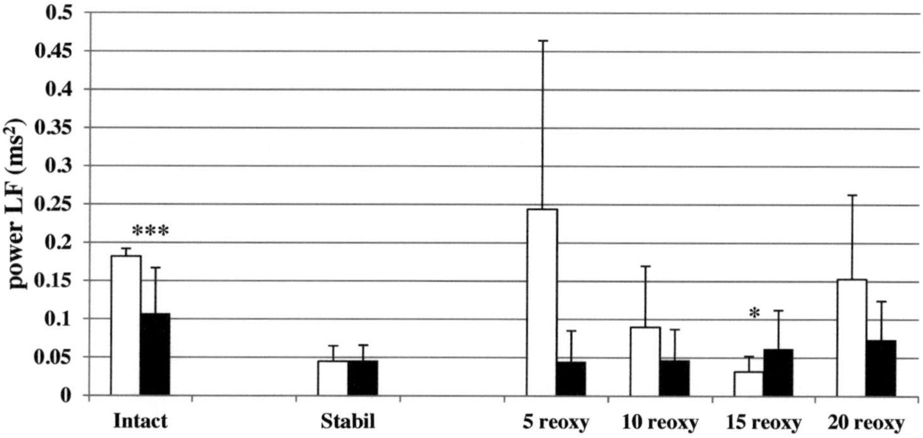

Figure 7. Mean ± SD values of the power LF in intact animals (Intact), after tracheotomy, thoracotomy and 5 min. stabilization (Stabil) and after 20 minute of artificial reoxygenation. Empty and black columns refer to light and dark parts of the day, respectively. The level of significance of differences between the light and dark part of the rat regime day is indicated by the symbol (* $p < 0{,}05$, *** $p < 0{,}001$).

LF and VLF components of the HRV did not show any regular and predictable changes in the duration of the experiment. Although significant LD differences was found in intact animals with longer duration in the light part, changes in these component practically did not depend on the LD cycle during the recovery of pulmonary ventilation (figure 7 and 8).

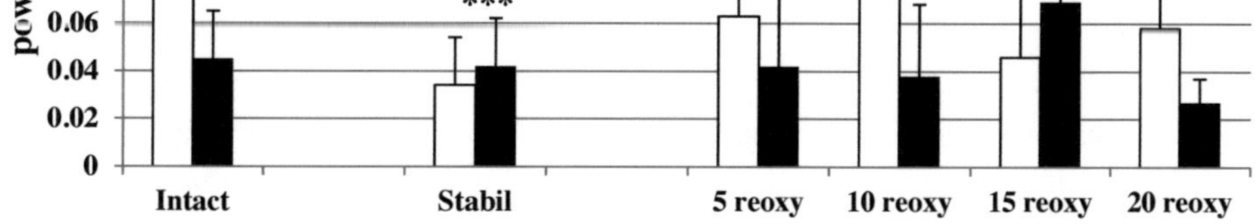

Figure 8. Mean ± SD values of the power VLF in intact animals (Intact), after tracheotomy, thoracotomy and 5 min. stabilization (Stabil) and after 20 minute of artificial reoxygenation. Empty and black columns refer to light and dark parts of the day, respectively. The level of significance of differences between the light and dark part of the rat regime day is indicated by the symbol (*** $p < 0{,}001$).

Ketamine/xylazine anaesthesia significantly increases the parasympathetic activity and decreases sympathetic and baroreceptor activity independently of the cycle of light and dark alternation. Under ketamine/xylazine anaesthesia, the RR interval duration preserves the significant LD differences resulting of the parasympathetic and baroreceptor activities as well in a dark (active) as well as in the light (inactive) mode on the rat day. Share of RR intervals is negligible to the sympathetic activity.

Reoxygenation the following immediately after the apnoic episode does not alter the relative abundance of the individual divissions of the ANS, but it is preserved the dominant parasympathetic activity (figure 9 and 10). During the light part of the day, the activity of the parasympathetic fluctuates randomly, but in a dark part of the day, we can see an increasing trend with time the duration of the reoxygenation. This tendency is comparable to the changes in the heart's electrical stability, which increases with the duration of the reoxygenation. Baroreceptor activity in the light part of the day fluctuates randomly, but in a dark part of the growing trend, which is probably associated with the predominant activity of the parasympathetic. Sympathetic activity during the reoxygenation shows no predictable changes in either of the lighted parts of the day.

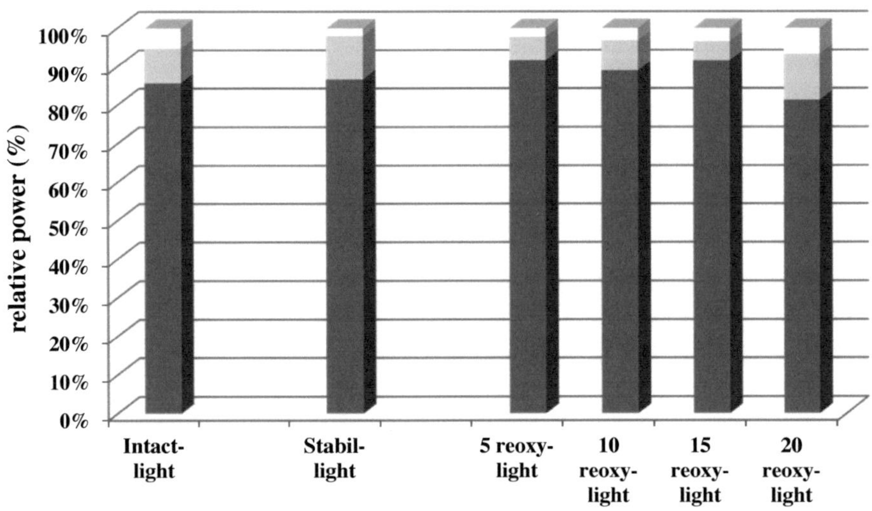

Figure 9. Relative power of the single components of HRV during the light part of the rat regime day. Black shadow – power HF, middle shadow – power LF and light shadow – power VLF.

In intact animals, correlation coefficients revealed that durations of RR intervals is influenced by parasympathetic and baroreceptor activities in both lighted parts of the day. Reoxygenation eliminated this dependence (table 1). We concluded that proarrythmogenic or antiarrhythmogenic effect of reoxygenation is probably connected with the changes in the parasympathetic activity and is dependent on the rat active or passive period in a ketamine/xylazine anaesthesia.

In ketamine/xylazine-anaesthetized rats, significant LD differences were preserved, in contrast to pentobarbital-anaesthetized rats (Svorc Jr. et al., 2013). Although the disruptive effect of ketamine on circadian rhythms has been described by others (Prudian et al., 1997; Pelissier et al., 1998), this effect was associated with modification of acrophase, amplitude or mesor, but without loss of daily rhythmicity. Ketamine/xylazine anaesthesia reduces heart rate in isolated rat heart preparations (Aronson and Hanno, 1978) and also in *in vivo* conditions (Salerno and vanTienhoven, 1976; Sapru and Krieger, 1979; Brown et al., 1994; Hoque et al., 1996; Maignan et al., 2000). It prolongs RR and QT intervals (Aronson and Hanno, 1978), decreases blood pressure (Sapru and Krieger, 1979), renal sympathetic activity and attenuates baroreflex sensitivity *in vivo* (Akine et al., 2001). On the other hand, Reid et al. (2003), described a stimulating effect on cardiac function during resuscitation. Unfortunately, in the above-mentioned studies, the clock time of the experiment was not reported, nor was the synchronization of animals to an LD regimen described.

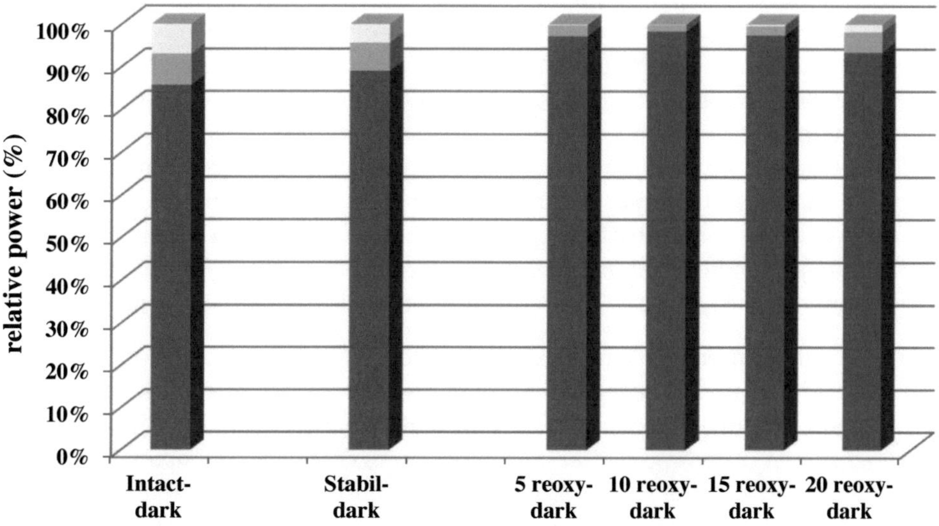

Figure 10. Relative power of the single components of HRV during the dark part of the rat regime day. Black shadow – power HF, middle shadow – power LF and light shadow – power VLF.

	Intact		Stabil		20 reoxy	
	light	dark	light	dark	light	dark
HF-RR	**r = 0,48**	**r = 0,44**	**r = 0,43**	r = 0,37	r = 0,05	**r = 0,5**
LF-RR	**r = 0,46**	**r = 0,45**	**r = 0,57**	**r = 0,56**	r = - 0,1	r = 0,1
VLF-RR	r = 0,19	r = 0,14	**r = 0,53**	r = 0,19	r = - 0,27	r = - 0,02

Table 1. Correlation coefficients between RR intervals duration and single parameters of HRV in the single experimental steps.

Results demostrate that ketamine/xylazine anaesthesia preferably increases parasympathetic activity and suppresses sympathetic and baroreceptor activity, resulting in marked bradycardia independently of the LD cycle. Presence of LD differences refers to the fact that this type of anaesthesia may be applicable in chronobiological studies. However, it may be problematic for cardiovascular research owing to serious bradycardia.

5. Conclusions

We concluded that the electrical myocardial properties are influenced by the changing cycles of light and darkness also in ketamine/xylazine anaesthesia.

- heart rate and electrical stability of the heart are significantly reduced by apneic episode regardless of the lighted period (proarrhythmogenic effect). Electrocardiographic parameters (PQ and QT interval) prolong with the duration of apneic episode regardless of the LD cycle. Possible cause of ventricular arrhythmias (ventricular arrhythmias originating from disorders of the impulse production and conduction or ventricular arrhythmias originating from an enlarged dispersion of refractory periods) probably depends not only on the duration of apneic episode, but also on the LD cycle. Short-term asphyxia increases vulnerability to the arrhythmias originating from disorders of the impulse production and conduction but does not disturb LD dependence. Long-term apneic episode, connected with more serious asphyxia continue increases vulnerability to this type of arrhythmias but independently on the LD cycle. The opposite situation is true of the QT interval.
- recovery of the pulmonary ventilation after apneic episodes can also contribute to heart rhythm disorders, but this is dependent upon the light (non-active)-dark (active) cycle. In the dark part of the day, the gradual decrease of the myocardial vulnerability is associated with the duration of reoxygenation (anti-arrhythmogenic effect) compared with the light part of the day, where the contrary tendency was observed (pro-arrhythmogenic effect). Reoxygenation disturbs LD differences in the heart rate as well as in QT interval duration, but recovers PQ interval duration to the pre-asphyxic values with preservation of the LD differences observed in intact animals.
- ketamine/xylazine anaesthesia increases parasympathetic activity, inhibits baroreceptor and sympathetic activity in the same way in both lighted periods. Dominant influence of parasympathetic autonomic nervous system was preserved during experiment. In these conditions, the heart is controled by the parasympathetic divission without the influence of the sympathetic autonomic nervous system.

Author details

Pavol Svorc[1,2], Ivana Bacova[1], Pavol Svorc, Jr.[2], Monika Novakova[1] and Alexander Marossy[1]

1 Department of Physiology, Medical Faculty, Safarik University, Kosice, Slovak Republic

2 Department of Physiology, Medical Faculty, Ostrava University, Ostrava, Czech Republic

References

[1] Akerstedt, T. & Wright, K.P., Jr. (2009). Sleep loss and fatigue in shift work and shift work disorder. *Sleep Medicine Clinics*, Vol. 4, No. 2, (June 2009), pp. 257-271, ISSN: 1556407X.

[2] Akine, A.; Suzuka, H.; Hayashida, Y. & Kato, Y. (2001). Effects of ketamine and propofol on autonomic cardiovascular function in chronically instrumented rats. *Autonomic Neuroscience-Basic & Clinical*, Vol. 87, No 2-3, (Mar 23 2001), pp. 201-208, ISSN: 1566-0702.

[3] Alva, N.; Palomeque, J. & Carbonell, T. (2006). Nitric oxide induced by ketamine/xylazine anesthesia maintains hepatic blood flow during hypothermia. *Nitric Oxide - Biology and Chemistry*, Vol. 15, No. 1, (Aug 2006), pp. 64-69, ISSN: 1089-8603

[4] Amitzur, G.; Schoels, W.; Visokovsky, A.; Lev-ran, V.; Novikov, I.; Mueller, M.; Kraft, P.; Kaplinsky, E. & Eldar, M. (2000). Role of sodium channels in ventricular fibrillation: A study in nonischemic isolated hearts. *Journal of Cardiovascular Pharmacology*, Vol. 36, No. 6, (Dec 2000), pp. 785-793, ISSN: 0160-2446.

[5] Arias, M.A. & Sanches, A.M. (2007). Obstructive sleep apnea and its relationship to cardiac arrhythmias. *Journal of Cardiovascular Electrophysiology*, Vol. 18, No. 9, (Sep 2007), pp. 1006-1014, ISSN: 1045-3873.

[6] Aronow, W.S. (2007). Cardiovascular manifestations seen in obstructive sleep apnea. *Comparative Therapy*, Vol. 33, No. 2, pp. 82-86, ISSN: 1559-1190

[7] Aronson, C.E. & Hanno, E.R.S. (1978). Effects of ketamine on the isolated perfused rat heart. *General Pharmacology*, Vol. 9, No. 4, (1978), pp. 249-255, ISSN: 0306-3623.

[8] Auger, R.R. & Morgenthaler, T.I. (2009). Jet lag and other sleep disorders relevant to the travel. *Travel Medicine and Infectious Diseases*, Vol.7, No. 2, (Mar 2009), pp. 60-68, ISSN: 1477-8939.

[9] Aydin, M.; Altin, R.; Ozeren, A.; Kart, L.; Bilge, M. & Unalacak, M. (2004). Cardiac autonomic activity in obstructive sleep apnea - Time-dependent and spectral analysis of heart rate variability using 24-hour holter electrocardiograms. *Texas Heart Institute Journal*, Vol. 31, No. 2, (2004), pp. 132-136, ISSN: 0730-2347.

[10] Aytemir, K.; Deniz, A.; Yavuz, B.; Demir, A.U.; Sahiner, L.; Ciftci, O.; Tokgozoglu, L.; Can, I.; Sahin, A. & Oto, A. (2007). Increased myocardial vulnerability and autonomic nervous system imbalance in obstructive sleep apnea syndrome. *Respiratory Medicine*, Vol. 101, No. 6, (Jun 2007), pp. 1277-1282, ISSN: 0954-6111.

[11] Bayram, N.A. & Diker, E. (2008). Obstructive sleep apnea syndrome and cardiac arrhythmias. *Turk Kardiyol Dern Ars*, Vol. 36, No. 1, pp. 44-50. PMID: 18453787 [PubMed - indexed for MEDLINE].

[12] Bacova, I.; Svorc, Jr. P.; Kundrik, M. & Fulton, B.L. (2010). Light-dark dependence of electrocardiographic changes during asphyxia and reoxygenation in a rat model. *Central European Journal of Medicine,* Vol. 5, No. 5, (Oct 2010), pp. 611-619, ISSN: 1895-1058.

[13] Billman, G.E.; Avendano, C.E.; Halliwill, J.R. & Burroughs, J.M. (1993). The effects of the ATP-dependent potassium channel antagonist, glyburide, on coronary blood-flow and susceptibility to ventricular fibrillation in unanesthetized dogs. *Journal of Cardiovascular Pharmacology,* Vol. 21, No. 2, (Feb 1993), pp. 197-204, ISSN: 0160-2446.

[14] Bishop, B.; Silva, G.; Krasney, J.; Nakano, H.; Roberts, A.; Farkas, G.; Rifkin, D. & Shucard, D. (2001). Ambient temperature modulates hypoxic - induced changes in rat body temperature and activity differentially. *American Journal of Physiology,* Vol. 280, No. 4, (Apr 2001), pp. R1190-R1196, ISSN: 0363-6119.

[15] Bosco, G.; Ionadi, A.; Panico, S.; Faralli, F.; Gagliardi, R.; Data, P. & Mortola, J.P. (2003). Effects of hypoxia on the circadian patterns in men. *High Altitude Medicine and Biology,* Vol. 4, No. 3, (Feb 2003), pp. 305-318, ISSN: 1527-0297.

[16] Bounhoure, J.P.; Galinier, M.; Didier, A. & Leophonte, P. (2005). Sleep apnea syndromes and cardiovascular disease. *Bulletin de l Academie Nationale de Medecine,* Vol. 189, No. 3, (Mar 2005), pp. 445-459, ISSN: 0001-4079.

[17] Brown, D.R.; Brown, L.V.; Patwardhan, A. & Randall, D.C. (1994). Sympathetic activity and blood-pressure are tightly coupled at 0,4 Hz in conscious rats. *American Journal of Physiology-Regulatory Integrative and Comparative Physiology,* Vol. 267, No. 5, (Nov 1994), pp. 1378-1384, ISSN: 0363-6119.

[18] Budhiraja, R. & Quan, S.F. (2005). Sleep-disordered breathing and cardiovascular health. *Current Opinion in Pulmonary Medicine,* Vol. 11, No. 6, (Nov 2005), pp. 501-506, ISSN: 1070-5287.

[19] Bugge, E.; Gamst, T.M.; Hegstad, A.C.; Andreassen, T. & Ytherus, K. (1997). Mepacrine protects the isolated rat heart during hypoxia and reoxagenation – but not by inhibition of phospholipase A2. *Basic Research in Cardiology,* Vol. 92, No. 1, (Feb 1997), pp. 17–24, ISSN: 0300-8428.

[20] Buggress, K.R. (1998). Central sleep apnoe and heart failure. *Respirology,* Vol. 3, No. 1, (Mar 1998), pp. 1-11. ISSN: 1440-1843, DOI: 10.1046/j.1440-1843.1998.d01-10.x

[21] Carmeliet, E. (1986). The slow inward current: non-voltage-clamp studies. In: *The slow invard current and cardiac arrhythmias,* Zipes, D.P.; Bailey, J.C.; Elharrar, V, pp. 97-110, Elsevier Science Publishers BV, ISBN: 978-94-009-8890-3, Hague/Boston/ London.

[22] Chen, C.C.; Chen, S.A.; Tai, C.T.; Kuo, T.B.J.; Chang, M.S. & Prystowsky, E.N. (2001). Hyperventilation facilitates induction of supraventricular tachycardia: A novel meth-

od and the possible mechanism. *Journal of Cardiovascular Electrophysiology*, Vol. 12, No. 11, (Nov 2001), pp. 1242-1246, ISSN: 1045-3873.

[23] Chowdhuri, S.; Crook, E.D.; Taylor, H.A. Jr. & Badr, M.S. (2007). Cardiovascular complications of respiratory diseases. *American Journal of the Medical Sciences*, Vol. 334, No. 5, (Nov 2007), pp. 361-380, ISSN: 0002-9629.

[24] Cope, D.K.; Impastato, W.K.; Cohen, M.V. & Downey, J.M. (1997). Volatile anesthetics protect the ischemic rabbit myocardium from infarction. *Anesthesiology*, Vol. 86, No. 3, (Mar 1997), pp. 699–709, ISSN: 0003-3022.

[25] Cutler, M.J.; Hamdam, A.L.; Hamdam, M.H.; Ramaswamy, K. & Smith, M.L. (2002). Sleep apnea: from the nose to the heart. *Jornal of the American Board of Family Medicine*, Vol. 15, No. 2, (Mar 2002), pp. 128-141, ISSN: 1558-7118.

[26] Daccarett, M.; Segerson, N.M.; Hamdan, A.L.; Hill, B. & Hamdan M.H. (2008). Relation of daytime bradyarrhythmias with high risk features of sleep apnea. *American Journal of Cardiology*, Vol. 101, No. 8, (Apr 15 2008), pp. 1147-1150, ISSN: 0002-9149.

[27] Daut, J.; Maierrudolph, W.; vonBeckerath, N.; Mehrke, G.; Gunther, K. & Goedel-Meinen, L. (1990). Hypoxic dilation of coronary-arteries is mediated by ATP-sensitive potassium channels. *Science*, Vol. 247,No. 4948, (Mar 16 1990), pp. 1341-1344, ISSN: 0036-8075.

[28] Dunai, A.; Musci, I.; Juhasz, J. & Novak, M. (2006). Obstructive sleep apnea and cardiovascular disease. *Orvosi Hetilap*, Vol. 147, No. 48, (2006-Dec-3), pp. 2303-2311, ISSN: 0030-6002.

[29] Farver, T.B.; Haskins, S.C. & Patz, J.D. (1986). Cardiopulmonary effects of acepromazine and of the subsequent administration of ketamine in the dog. *American Journal of Veterinary Research*, Vol. 47, No. 3, (Mar 1986), pp. 631-635, ISSN: 0002-9645.

[30] Foster, G.T.; Vaziri, N.D. & Sassoon, C.S. (2001). Respiratory alkalosis. *Respiratory Care*, Vol. 46, No. 4, (2001-Apr), pp. 384-391, ISSN: 0020-1324.

[31] Froldi, G.; Pandolfo, L.; Chinellato, A.; Ragazzi, E.; Caparrotta, L. & Fassina, G. (1994). Protection of atrial function in hypoxia by high potassium concentration. *General Pharmacology*, Vol. 25, No. 3, (May 1994), pp. 401-407, ISSN: 0306-3623.

[32] Gami, A.S.; Howard, D.E.; Olson, E.J. & Somers, V.K. (2005). Day-night pattern of sudden death in obstructive sleep apnea. *New England Journal of Medicine*, Vol. 352, No. 12, (Mar 2005), pp. 1206-1214, ISSN: 0028-4793.

[33] Gilpin, E.A.; Hjalmarson, A. &, Ross, J. (1990). Subgroups of patients with atypical circadian patterns of symptom oset in acute myocardial infardction. *American Journal of Cardiology*, Vol. 66, No. 16, (Nov 6 1990), pp. 7G-11G, ISSN: 0002-9149.

[34] Gresova, S.; Tomori, Z.; Kurpas, M.; Marossy, A.; Vrbenska, A.; Kundrik, M. & Donic, V. (2009). Blood pressure increase detected by ambulatory monitoring correlates

with hypoxemia reflecting sleep apnea severity. *Central European Journal of Medicine*, Vol. 4, No. 2, (Jun 2009), pp. 222-232, ISSN: 1895-1058.

[35] Griffiths, E,J.; Ocampo, C.J.; Savage, J.S.; Stern, M.D. & Silverman, H.S. (2000). Protective effects of low and high doses of cyclosporin A against reoxygenation injury in isolated rat cardiomyocytes are associated with differrential effects on mitochondrial calcium levels. *Cell Calcium*, Vol. 27, No. 2, (Feb 2000), pp. 87-95, ISSN: 0143-4160.

[36] Gunez, Y.; Tuncer, M.; Guntekin, U.; Akdag, S. & Gumrukcuoglu, H.A. (2008). Lack of diurnal variation of P-wave and QT dispersions in patients with heart failure. *PACE – Pacing and Clinical Electrophysiology*, Vol. 31, No. 8, (Aug 2008), pp. 974-978, ISSN: 0147-8389.

[37] Hayashida, Y.; Hirakawa, H.; Nakamura, T. & Maeda, M. (1996). Chemoreceptors in autonomic responses to hypoxia in conscious rats. In: *Frontiers in Arterial Chemoreception*, Zapata, P.; Eyzaguirre, C. & Torrance, R.W., pp. 439-442, Plenum Press, ISBN: 0-306-45490-4, New York.

[38] Henry, R.; Casto, R. & Printz, M.P. (1990) Diurnal cardiovascular patterns in spontaneously hypertensive and Wistar-Kyoto rats. *Hypertension*, Vol. 16, No. 4, (Oct 1990), pp. 422-428, ISSN: 0194-911X.

[39] Hinojosa-Laborde, C. & Mifflin, S.W. (2005). Sex differences in blood pressure response to intermittent hypoxia in rats. *Hypertension*, Vol. 46, No. 4, (Oct 2005), pp. 1016-1021, ISSN: 0194-911X.

[40] Hsu, W.H.; Bellin, S.I.; Dellmann, H.D.; Habil, V. & Hanson, C.E. (1986). Xylazine-ketamine – induced anesthesia in rats and its antagonism by yohimbine. *Journal of the American Veterinary Association*, Vol. 189, No. 9, (Nov 1 1986), pp. 1040–1043, ISSN: 0003-1488.

[41] Hoque, A.M.; Marczin, N.; Catravas, J.D. & Fuchs, L.C. (1996). Anesthesia with sodium pentobarbital enhances lipopolysaccharide-induced cardiovascular dysfunction in rats. *Shock*, Vol. 6, No. 5, (Nov 1996), pp. 365- 370, ISSN: 1073-2322.

[42] Kaplan, J.L.; Gao, E.; deGaravilla, L.; Victain, M.; Minczak, B. & Dalsey, W.C. (2003). Adenosine A1 antagonism attenuates atropine-resistant hypoxic bradycardia in rats. *Academic Emergency Medicine*, Vol. 10, No. 9, (Sep 2003), pp. 923-930, ISSN: 1069-6563.

[43] Kuniyoshi, F.H.S.; Garcia-Touchard, A.; Gami, A.S.; Romero-Corral, A.; van der Walt, C.; Pusalavidyasagar, S.; Kara, T.; Caples, S.M.; Pressman, G.S.; Vasquez, E.C.; Lopez-Jimenez, F. & Somers, V.K. (2008). Day-night variation of acute myocardial infarction in obstructive sleep apnea. *Journal of the American College Cardiolology*, Vol. 52, No. 5, (Jul 2008), pp. 343-346, ISSN: 0735-1097.

[44] Leone, R. Jr. & Merrill, G.F. (1995). Inhibition of adenosine deaminase and administration of adenosine increase hypoxia induced ventricular ectopy. *Basic Research in Cardiology*, Vol. 90, No. 3, (May-Jun 1995), pp. 234-239, ISSN: 0300-8428.

[45] Lubbe, W.F.; Bricknell, O.L. & Marzagao, C. (1975). Ventricular fibrillation threshold and vulnerable period in the isolated perfused rat heart. *Cardiovascular Research*, Vol. 9, No. 5, (Sep 1975), pp. 613-620, ISSN: 0008-6363.

[46] Maignan, E.; Dong, W.X.; Legrand, M.; Safar, M. & Cuche, J.L. (2000). Sympathetic activity in the rat: effects of anaesthesia on noradrenaline kinetics. *Journal of the Autonomic Nervous System*, Vol. 80, No. 1-2, (Apr 12 2000), pp. 46-51, ISSN: 0165-1838.

[47] Morita, Y.; Murakami, T.; Iwase, T.; Nagal, K.; Nawada, R.; Kouchi, I.; Akao, M. & Sasayama, S. (1997). K_{ATP} channels contribute to the cardioprotection of preconditioning independent of anaesthetics in rabbit hearts. *Journal of Molecular and Cellular Cardiology*, Vol. 29, No. 4, (Apr 1997), pp. 1267–1276, ISSN: 0022-2828.

[48] Mortola, J.P. & Seifert, E.L. (2000). Hypoxic depression of circadian rhythms in adult rats. *Journal of Applied Physiology*. Vol. 88, No. 2, (Feb 2000), pp. 365-368, ISSN: 8750-7587.

[49] Mortola, J.P. (2007). Hypoxia and circadian patterns. *Respiratory Physiology & Neurobiology*, Vol. 158, No. 2-3, (Sep 30 2007), pp. 274-279, ISSN: 1569-9048.

[50] Mubagwa, K.; Kaplan, P. & Flameng, W. (1997). The effects of ryanodine on calcium uptake by the sarcoplasmic reticulum of ischemic and reperfused rat myocardium. *Fundamental and Clinical Pharmacology*, Vol. 11, No. 4, (1997), pp. 315–321, ISSN: 0767-3981.

[51] Mukai, M.; Terada, H.; Sugiyama, S.; Satoh, H. & Hayashi, H. (2000). Effects of a selective inhibitor of Na^+/Ca^{2+} exchange, KB-R7943, on reoxygenation – induced injuries in guinea pig papillary muscles. *Journal of Cardiovascular Pharmacology*, 2000, Vol. 36, No. 3, (Sep 2000), pp. 416-416, ISSN: 0160-2446.

[52] Nishimura, M.; Tanaka, H.; Homma, N.; Matsuzawa, T. & Watanabe, Y. (1989). Ionic mechanisms of the depression of automaticity and conduction in the rabbit atrioventricular node caused by hypoxia or metabolic inhibition and protective action of glucose and valine. *American Journal of Cardiology*, Vol. 64, No. 20, (Dec 1989), pp. J24–J28, ISSN: 0002-9149.

[53] Noda, A.; Yasuma, F.; Okada, T.; Yokota, M. (1988). Circadian rhythm of autonomic activity in patients with obstructive sleep apnea syndrome. *Clinical Cardiology*, Vol. 21, No. 4, (Apr 1998), pp. 271-276, ISSN: 0160-9289.

[54] Noma, A. & Shibasaki, T. (1985). Membrane current through adenosine-triphosphate-regulated potassium channels in guinea-pig ventricular cells. *Journal of Physiology-London*, Vol. 363, No. Jun, (1985), pp. 463-480, ISSN: 0022-3751.

[55] Opie, L.H.; Nathar, D. & Lubbe, W.F. (1979). Biochemical aspects of arrhythmogenesis and ventricular fibrillation. *American Journal of Cardiology*, Vol. 43, No. 1, (Jan 1979), pp. 131–148, ISSN: 0002-9149.

[56] Overgaard, J.; Gesser, H.; Wang, T.; Tribute, T.O. & Lutz, P.L. (2007). Cardiac performance and cardiovascular regulation during anoxia/hypoxia in freshwater turtles.

Journal of Experimental Biology, Vol. 210, (May 2007), pp. 1687-1699, ISSN: 1477-9145, doi:10.1242/jeb.001925.

[57] Parish, J.M. & Somers, V.K. (2004). Obstructive sleep apnea and cardiovascular disease. *Mayo Clinic Proceedings*, Vol. 79, No. 8, (Aug 2004), pp. 1036-1046, ISSN: 0025-6196.

[58] Park, D.H.; Shin, C.J.; Hong, S.C.; Yu, J.; Ryu, S.H.; Kim, E.J.; Shin, H.B. & Shin, B.H. (2008). Correlation between the severity of obstructive sleep apnea and heart rate variability indices. *Journal of Korean Medical Science*, Vol. 23, No. 2, (Apr 2008), pp. 226-231, ISSN: 1011-8934.

[59] Patel, N. & Rosen, I. (2007). Sleep apnea and cardiovascular disease: Association, causation, and implication. *Clinical Pulmonary Medicine*, Vol. 14, No. 4, (July 2007), pp. 225-231. doi: 10.1097/CPM.0b013e3180cac6d8

[60] Pelissier, A.L.; Gantenbein, M.; Prudian, F. & Bruguerolle, B. (1998). Influence of general anaethetics on circadian rhythms of heart rate, body temperature and locomotor activity in rats. *Sciences et Techniques de l Animal de Laboratoire*, Vol. 23, No. 2, (1998), pp. 91-98, ISSN: 0339-722X.

[61] Perchenet, L. & Kreher, P. (1995). Mechanical and electrophysiological effects of preconditioning in isolated ischemic/reperfused rat heart. *Journal of Cardiovascular Pharmacology*, Vol. 26, No. 5, (Nov 1995), pp. 831–840, ISSN: 0160-2446.

[62] Portaluppi, F. & Hermida, R.C. (2007). Circadian rhythms in cardiac arrhythmias and opportunities for their chronotherapy. *Advanced Drug Delivery Reviews*, Vol. 59, No. 9-10, (Aug 31 2007), pp. 940-951, ISSN: 0169-409X.

[63] Prudian, F.; Gantenbein, M.; Pelissier A.L.; Attolini, L. & Bruguerolle, B. (1997). Daily rhythms of heart rate, temperature and locomotor activity are modified by anaesthetics in rats: A telemetric study. *Naunyn–Schmiedebergs Archives Pharmacology*, Vol. 355, No. 6, (Jun 1997), pp. 774-778, ISSN: 0028-1298.

[64] Reid, K.H.; Paskitti, M.; Guo, S.Z.; Schmeizer, T. & Iyer, V. (2003). Experience with ketamine and sodium pentobarbital as anesthetics in a rat model of cardiac arrest and resuscitation. *Resuscitation*, Vol. 57, No. 2, (May 2003), pp. 201-210, ISSN: 0300-9572.

[65] Richardson, G.S. (2005). The human circadian system in normal and disordered sleep. *Journal of Clinical Psychiatry*, Vol. 66, suppl 9, (2005), pp. 7-9, ISSN: 0160-6689.

[66] Roche, F.; Xuong, A.N.T.; Court-Fortune, I.; Costes, F.D.; Pichot, V.; Duverney, D.; Vergnon, J.M.; Gaspoz, J.M. & Barthelemy, J.C. (2003). Relationship among the severity of sleep apnea syndrome, cardiac arrhythmias, and autonomic imbalance. *PACE-Pacing and Clinical Electrophysiology*, Vol. 26, No. 3, (Mar 2003), pp. 669-677, ISSN: 0147-8389.

[67] Salerno, A. & van Tienhoven, A. (1976). The effect of ketamine on heart rate, respiration rate and EEG of white leghorn hens. *Comparative Biochemistry and Physiology. C: Comparative Pharmacology*, Vol. 55, No. 1, (1976), pp. 69-75, ISSN: 0306-4492.

[68] Sanguinetti, M.C.; Scott, A.L.; Zingaro, G.J. & Siegl. P.K.S. (1988). BRL-34915 (Cromakalim) activates ATP-sensitive K^+ current in cardiac-muscle. *Proceedings of the National Academy of Sciences of the United States of America*, Vol. 85, No. 21, (Nov 1988), pp. 8360-8364, ISSN: 0027-8424.

[69] Sapru, H.N. & Krieger, A.J. (1979). Cardiovascular and respiratory effects of some anesthetics in the decerebrate rat. *European Journal of Pharmacology*, Vol. 53, No. 2, (1979-Jan-1), pp. 151-158, ISSN: 0014-2999.

[70] Sawanobori, T.; Adaniya, H.; Yukisada, H. & Hiraoka, M. (1995). Role for ATP – sensitive K^+ channel in the development of A – V block during hypoxia. *Journal of Molecular and Cellular Cardiology*, Vol. 27, No. 1, (Jan 1995), pp. 647–657, ISSN: 0022-2828.

[71] Schulz, R.; Grebe, M.; Eisele, H.J.; Mayer, K.; Weissmann, N. & Seeger, W. (2006). Obstructive sleep apnea-related cardiovascular disease. *Medizinische Klinik*, Vol. 101, No. 4, (Apr 15 2006), pp. 321-327, ISSN: 0723-5003.

[72] Shinmura, K.; Tani, M.; Suganuma, Y.; Hasegawa, H.; Ebihara, Y.; Nakamura, Y. & Asakura, Y. (1997). Effects of alpha(1)-adrenoreceptor subtype blockade on ischemia – reperfusion injury. *Japanese Circulation Journal*, Vol. 61, No. 11, (Nov 1997), pp. 927–935, ISSN: 0047-1828.

[73] Sumitra, M.; Manikandan, P.; Rao, K.V.K.; Nayeem, M.; Manohar, B.M. & Puvanakrishnan, R. (2004). Cardiorespiratory effects of diazepam-ketamine, xylazine-ketamine and thiopentone anesthesia in male Wistar rats – A comparative analysis. *Life Science*, Vol. 75, No.15, (Aug 27 2004), pp. 1887-1896, ISSN: 0024-3205.

[74] Svorc, P.; Wilk, P.; Murár, J. Podlubny I.; Kujanik S.; Bracokova I. & Murin M. (1994). Circadian rhythm of the ventricular fibrillation threshold in female Wistar rats. *Physiological Research*, Vol. 43, No. 6, (Sep 1994), pp. 355–358, ISSN: 0369-9463.

[75] Svorc, P.; Podlubny, I.; Kujanik, S. & Bracokova, I. (1997). 24h rhythm of the vetricular fibrillation threshold during normal and hypoventilation in female Wistar rats. *Chronobiology International*, Vol. 14, No. 4, (Feb 1997), pp. 363–370, ISSN: 0742-0528.

[76] Svorc, P.; Bracokova, I. & Podlubny, I. (2000). Relation of ventricular fibrillation threshold to heart rate during normal ventilation and hypoventilation in female Wistar rats: A chronophysiological study. *Physiological Research,* Vol. 49, No. 6, (Mar 2000), pp. 711 –719, ISSN 0862-8408.

[77] Svorc, P.; Bracokova, I.; Bacova, I. & Svorcova, E. (2009). Acid-base balance and artifitial controlled ventilation in Wistar rats, Chronobiological view. *Abstract book from The third International Congress of Applied Chronobiology and Chronomedicine*, Akko Israel, pp. 67.

[78] Svorc, P. Jr.; Svorc, P. & Fulton, B.L. (2011). Chronobiological aspects of reoxygenation impact on the heart rhythm disorders in Wistar rat model. *Trends in Comp Biochem Physiol*, Vol. 15, pp. 55-61, ISSN: 0972-4540.

[79] Svorc, P.; Marossy, A.; Svorc, P. Jr; Gresova, S.; Buzga, M. & Fulton, B.J. (2012). Chronobiological aspects of the heart rhythm disorders at the change of pulmonary ventilation in rat model. In: *Cardiac arrhythmias. New Considerations*, Breijo-Marquez, F.R, pp. 193-226, InTech, ISBN: 978-953-51-0126-0, Rijeka, Croatia

[80] Svorc, P. Jr.; Bacova, I.; Svorc, P. & Buzga, M. (2013). Autonomic nervous system under ketamine/xylazine and pentobarbital anaesthesia in a Wistar rat model: Chronobiological view. *Prague Medical Report*, Vol. 114, No. 2, (Apr. 2013), pp. 72-80, ISSN 1214-6994.

[81] Tukek, T.; Yildiz, P.; Atilgan, D.; Tuzcu, V.; Eren, M.; Erk, O.; Demirel, S.; Akkaya, V.; Dilmener, M. & Korkut, F. (2003). Effect of diurnal variability of heart rate on development of arrhythmia in patients with chronic obstructive pulmonary disease. *International Journal of Cardiology*, Vol. 88, No. 2-3, (Apr 2003), pp. 199-206, ISSN: 0167-5273.

[82] Waterhouse, J.; Witte, K.; Huser, L.; Nevill, A.; Atkinson, G.; Reilly, T. & Lemmer, B. (2000). Sensitivity of heart rate and blood pressure to spontaneous activity in transgenic rats. *Biological Rhythm Research*, Vol. 31, No. 2, (Apr 2000), pp. 146-159, ISSN: 0929-1016.

[83] Wolleben, C.D.; Sanguinetti, M.C. & Siegl, P.K.S. (1989). Influence of ATP-sensitive potassium channel modulators on ischemia-induced fibrillation in isolated rat hearts. *Journal of Molecular and Cellular Cardiology*, Vol. 21, No. 8, (Aug 1989), 783-788, ISSN: 0022-2828.

[84] Xu, J.; Wang, L.; Hurt, C.M. & Pelleg, A. (1994). Endogenous adenosine does not activate ATPsensitive pottasium channels in the hypoxic guinea pig ventricle in vivo. *Circulation*, Vol. 89, No. 3, (Mar 1994), pp. 1209-1216, ISSN: 1524-4539.

[85] Yamashita, J.; Nomura, M.; Uehara, K.; Nakaya, Y.; Uemura, E.; Iga, A.; Sawa, Y.; Nishikado, A.; Saito, K. & Ito, S. (2004). Influence of sleep apnea on autonomic nervous activity and QT dispersion in patients with essential hypertension and old myocardial infarction. *Journal of Electrocardiology*, Vol. 37, No. 1, (Jan 2004), pp. 31-40, doi: 10.1016/j.jelectrocard.2003.10.009

Chapter 3

Detection, Tracking and Related Costs of Ablation Catheters in the Treatment of Cardiac Arrhythmias

Pascal Fallavollita

Additional information is available at the end of the chapter

http://dx.doi.org/10.5772/57424

1. Introduction

The adjective *'cardiac'* signifies *'related to the heart'* and it originates from the Greek word *'kardia'* meaning *'heart'*. The human heart is a muscular pump roughly the size of a fist. It pumps blood continuously through the circulatory system. The average human heart will beat at 72 beats per minute, and beat 2.5 billion times during a 66 year lifespan. Further, the heart pumps an average 5.2 liters of blood per minute. It weighs approximately 250 to 300 grams in females and 300 to 350 grams in males [1].

The heart's electrical system includes three parts (see Figure 1):

1. *S-A node* (sinoatrial node)– known as the heart's natural pacemaker, the S-A node has special cells that create the electricity that makes your heart beat.
2. *A-V node* (atrioventricular node)– the bridge between the atria and ventricles. Electrical signals pass from the atria down to the ventricles through the A-V node.
3. *His-Purkinje system*– carries the electrical signals throughout the ventricles via conduction pathways to make them contract.

Severe disorders of the heart rhythm can lead to sudden cardiac death (SCD), which is a sudden and unexpected death. Not to be confused with heart attacks which occur because of coronary artery blockage, sudden cardiac death happens when the electrical system of the heart becomes very irregular leading the heart to beat dangerously fast. At the outset of such a scenario, the greatest concern becomes blood flow to the brain being reduced, and unless treated rapidly patient death ensues.

In 2012, a review of the epidemiology of SCD was disseminated [3]. For brevity, we provide only a short summary of its highlights. In the United States alone, the incidence rate ranges

INTECH
open science | open minds

© 2014 Fallavollita; licensee InTech. This is a paper distributed under the terms of the Creative Commons Attribution License (http://creativecommons.org/licenses/by/3.0), which permits unrestricted use, distribution, and reproduction in any medium, provided the original work is properly cited.

between 180,000 and 450,000 cases annually [3, 4]. These estimates vary owing to differences in SCD definitions and surveillance methods [3, 5]. Prospective studies using multiple centers within the United States [3, 6-7], Netherlands [3, 8], Ireland [3, 9] and China [3, 10] showed SCD rates ranging from 50 to 100 per 100,000 general populations. From these, it is clear that the overall burden in the population remains high. Improvements in primary and secondary prevention have resulted in substantial declines in overall coronary heart disease (CHD) mortality over the past 30 years [3, 11-12], whereas SCD rates specifically have declined to a lesser extent [3, 13-16]. SCD still accounts for 50% of all CHD deaths and up to 20% of all deaths [3, 17]. For some segments of the population, rates are not decreasing and may actually be increasing [3, 14, 18]. As such, SCD prevention represents a major opportunity to further reduce mortality from CHD [3].

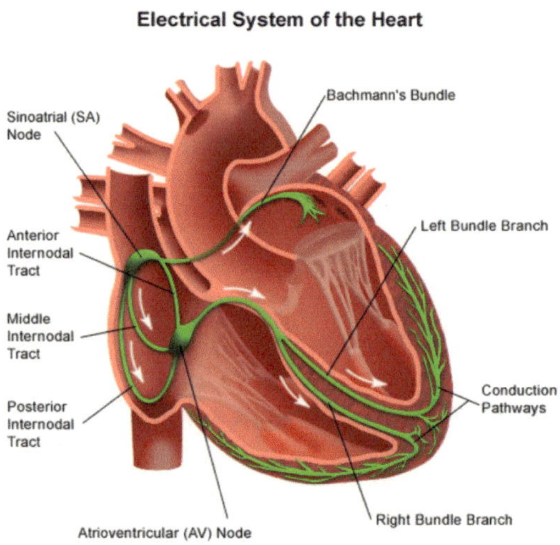

Figure 1. The electrical activity of the heart – image taken from [2].

i. Radiofrequency catheter ablation

Cardiac arrhythmias have been linked to SCD and the handling of these has been facilitated by the ability to definitively treat many patients with radiofrequency (RF) catheter ablation. Two very common arrhythmias treated are atrial fibrillation (AF) and ventricular tachycardia (VT). The first originates by impulses beginning and spreading through the atria, competing for a chance to travel through the AV node. The heart rhythm becomes disorganized, rapid, and irregular resulting in loss of coordinated atrial contraction. On the other hand, VT is a rapid rhythm originating from the lower chambers of the heart. It prevents the heart from filling adequately with blood, thereby less blood is able to pump through the body. VT is considered a more serious arrhythmia.

Authors in [19] provide an excellent review on the history and evolution of RF ablation. Catheter ablation with direct current from a standard external defibrillator began to supersede surgery in the 1980's. A shock was delivered between the distal catheter electrode and a

http://dx.doi.org/10.5772/57424

cutaneous surface electrode [19]. However, this high-voltage discharge was difficult to control and could cause tissue damage. As clinicians became more skilled and electrophysiological mapping improved, direct current (DC) ablation was used to treat cases of Wolff-Parkinson-White, ventricular tachycardia and atrial tachycardia [19, 20-25]. By the 1990's, radiofrequency energy had supplanted direct current [19, 26] since there was high incidence of complications associated with the high-energy discharge. In addition to this, RF ablation could be performed on conscious patients [19, 27-29].

Today, catheter ablation procedures are performed in an electrophysiology laboratory. RF electrode catheters are most commonly inserted percutaneously into the femoral veins and orientated within the heart to allow pacing stimulation and intracardiac electrical signal recording at key sites: such as the right atrium, right ventricle, the area of the His bundle or the coronary sinus [19, 30]. The efficacy of catheter ablation is highly dependent on accurate identification of the site of origin of the arrhythmia. Once this site has been identified, an ablation catheter (typically 7-11 French in size, see Figure 2) is positioned in direct contact with it and radiofrequency energy is delivered to ablate it. After one minute, a lesion of 5-mm depth is formed, which is enough to destroy the full thickness of the atrial myocardium in that location [19, 30].

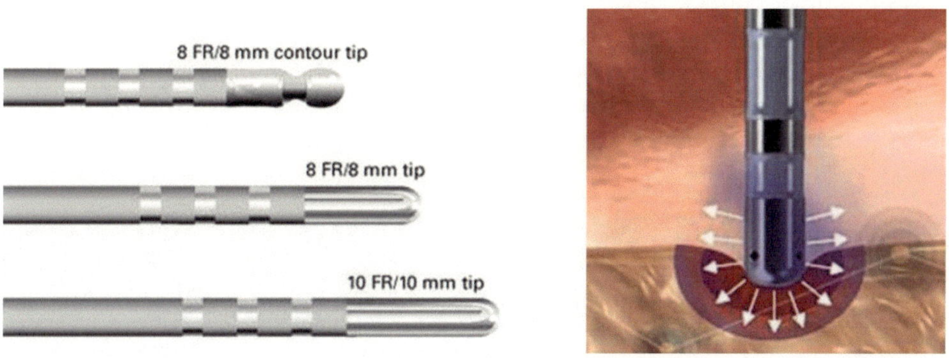

Figure 2. *Left*) Radiofrequency cardiac ablation catheters of different sizes - image taken from [36]. (*Right*) The catheter tip delivers the bursts of high energy waves that destroy the abnormal areas image taken from [37].

Current ablation systems allow for temperature monitoring and control [31]. These are valuable tools during RF ablation procedures as they: (i) provide important information regarding the adequacy of tissue heating, (ii) minimize the development of coagulum, and (iii) maximize the lesion size. Newer technical modifications, such as a larger distal electrode and saline cooling of this electrode, have helped to minimize impedance rises and allow creation of larger and deeper lesions [19, 32–35].

ii. Radiation exposure

Catheter ablation is often a long procedure requiring fluoroscopy exposure. RF ablation usually can routinely be accomplished with <20 min of fluoroscopy for most arrhythmias [19]. In 2012, a task force led by prominent cardiologists defined guidelines and recommendations for ablation procedural techniques, patient management and follow-up [38]. One concern raised was that an important complication of ablation is the delayed effect of the radiation received by the patients which yield [39] malignancy, and genetic abnormalities [40]. Many of the described studies in [38] demonstrated that catheter ablation of atrial fibrillation required significantly greater fluoroscopy duration and radiation exposure than simpler catheter ablation procedures. Thus, increasing availability and familiarity of electrophysiologists with 3D mapping systems [41] may significantly reduce fluoroscopy time. The task force recommendation is that this can only be achieved by an awareness of the importance of reducing fluoroscopy time, and therefore radiation exposure, by the operator. Although it is hypothesized that use of remote 3D navigation systems will reduce radiation exposure to patients and operators, this remained unproven until recently [38].

iii. 3D Mapping systems

An overview of cardiac mapping technologies is presented in [42]. The use of non-fluoroscopic techniques, using either magnetic or electrical fields for mapping of catheter position, has reduced fluoroscopy time and radiation dose to both patient and staff.

The common mapping technologies that combine 3D anatomy and electrophysiological data are: *CARTO* and *CARTOMerge* (Biosense Webster), *NavX* (St.Jude Medical), and *RPM* (Cardiac Pathways-Boston Scientific). Other technologies that provide continuous data of all electrophysiogical events include *Ensite 3000* (St. Jude Medical) and *Basket* (Cardiac Pathways-EP Technologies) [43-44]. More sophisticated mapping technologies that involve the fusion of imaging modalities (i.e. using preoperative MRI/CT, to fluoroscopy) are also discussed [45]. Two sample visualizations of the above technologies are seen in Figure 3.

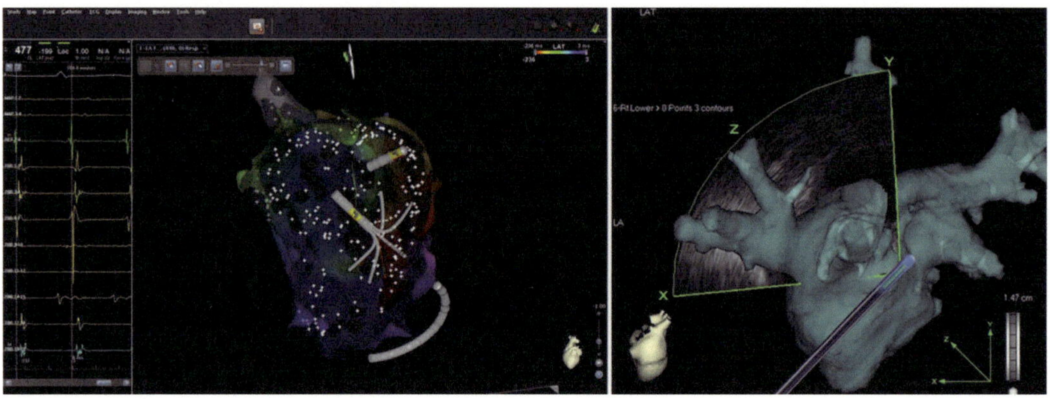

Figure 3. BioSense Webster has recently released (*left*) a multi-electrode mapping version of its 3D cardiac mapping system, and (*right*) a platform to merge ultrasound data of the heart [37].

An alternative technology is the intracardiac echocardiography (ICE) which has become the imaging modality of choice in many interventional settings primarily due to its flexibility and ease of use. The most commonly used ICE transducer is the *ACUNAV* (Siemens Medical Solution) which provides real-time visualization of structural anatomy. Another advantage of

http://dx.doi.org/10.5772/57424

such a transducer is that it delivers precise information about catheter position and adjacent structures. The first report of the various uses of ICE in atrial fibrillation is outlined in [42]. These include but are not limited to: (i) facilitating transseptal puncture, (ii) assisting catheter positioning prior to ablation, and (iii) identifying pulmonary vein structure. Also reported is the efficacy of ICE during the treatment of ventricular tachycardia [46]. Here, ICE is used to monitor catheter position and stability, and additionally is used to visualize the aortic cusp region. Lastly, registration between ICE and a 3D reconstruction of the left atria, performed using rotational fluoroscopy, is reported and shown to be an alternative technique to support atrial fibrillation ablation [47].

Robotic cardiac catheter ablation has been recently developed to eliminate potential errors in catheter manipulation. Also, the use of robots could systematically decrease clinician fatigue and fluoroscopy exposure. Some electrophysiologists agree that areas between mitral valves and pulmonary veins are typically difficult to reach and position correctly the mapping catheter. Robotics can thus provide more accuracy in these cases. Yet, initial studies show complications can occur at about the same rate as manual ablation. Currently there are two robotic systems – the *Stereotaxis Magnetic Navigation System* (Stereotaxis, Inc.) and the *Hansen Sensei Robotic Catheter System* (Hansen Medical). Both systems allow the physician to perform the mapping and ablation procedure while sitting in a control room remote from the patient [48]. Ongoing robotic developments use a magnetic tracking device to track the distal part of the ablation catheter in real time, and a master-slave robot-assisted system for actuation of a steerable catheter [49].

iv. Hospital induced costs

In 2013, an exhaustive study was released that evaluated the cost of special equipment chosen by physicians to perform cardiac ablations [50]. More specifically, the costs associated with the treatment of atrial fibrillation procedures were investigated. A synopsis of the relevant costs follows.

Cost of mapping technology: the 5-year cost for the mapping systems and maintenance is $375,000 (Biosense Webster Carto 3) and $495,000 (St. Jude EnSite Velocity). Phased array ICE catheters use standard ultrasound machines. The rotational ultrasound catheter (Ultra ICE, Boston Scientific, Natick, MA, USA) requires a special machine (iLab®) with a 5-year cost of $131,400. Lastly, the 5-year cost ranged from $33,000–$67,000 for the traditional RF generators [50].

Cost of catheters: Catheters compatible with the St. Jude Ensite Velocity system ranged from $1,500–$1,900, and the special navigation catheters required by Carto 3 cost $2,800–$3,000. The lowest cost ICE catheter is the Boston Scientific Ultra ICE™ rotational catheter costing $1,050. The most expensive are the phased-array catheters costing $2,640–$2,800. Although the rotational ICE catheter costs $1,590 less than the phased array, it requires a separate ultrasound processor (iLab®); therefore, it takes 82.6 cases to begin saving on each rotational ICE catheter [50].

Cost of Robotic Systems: The manufacturer's list price for the Stereotaxis NIROBE Robotic magnetic navigation system (MNS) is $2,875,000 with an annual maintenance contract of

$104,000 per year for a total 6-year cost of $3,395,000. Assuming 200 patient cases per year, the robotic MNS costs $2,829 per case. It requires a disposable $1,200/case ablation catheter advancement system and $250/case circular mapping catheter drive. The system requires special catheters which cost $3,590 including cables and irrigation tubing and can only utilize the Carto 3 mapping system. The lowest- and highest-cost scenarios for a MNS ablation are $12,261 and $15,464. These costs for MNS ablation are 84.7 and 133 % higher than the lowest-cost RF equipment [50].

Cost of The Medtronic Arctic Front® cryoballoon cost is $6,500.The costs of a cryoballoon ablation with focal cryoablation touch-up for the lowest- or highest-cost scenarios is similar to that for the balloon-only ablation, but requires the addition of a Freezor® MAX focal cryoablation catheter for $3,095. The lowest cost estimate requires repeated removal of the cryoballoon and insertion of the focal ablation catheter through the same sheath. The highest-cost estimate assumes the addition of a variable-diameter circular mapping catheter used independently of the cryoballoon through a steerable sheath. The total lowest and highest costs of $15,942 and $22,284 were 140 % and 236 % higher than the lowest-cost RF ablation [50].

The conclusions of the study [50] are that hospitals and clinicians have many choices of ablation equipment. These equipment costs ranged from $6,637 to $22,284 per case. In the end, the development of more expensive technologies should demonstrate an increase in the efficiency of cardiac ablation procedures as well as positive patient outcomes.

2. Detection and tracking of cardiac ablation catheters

There are several reasons as to why detecting and tracking the position of ablation catheters relative to the patient anatomy is important. They are related to interventional guidance aspects: (i) accounting for heart motion compensation, (ii) easing positioning & navigation during cardiac ablation, (iii) planning the ablation procedure by (iv) registration to preoperative data such as CT and MRI. To achieve detection and tracking, there are two primary options available: (a) hardware solutions that include mechanical and optical systems or the previously mentioned mapping systems, and (b) software and image-based solutions that make use of intraoperative images such as X-ray fluoroscopy.

We observe notable differences when comparing mapping systems with image-based solutions. First, although mapping solutions are expensive, they provide high accuracy and robustness and their clinical usage is getting popular. However, there is a notable learning curve for clinicians to get used to this technology. As for image-guided solutions, these require dealing with high data variation and involve the acquisition of a large amount of X-ray images. Their usage is still very limited since there is a high performance requirement for a practical clinical solution.

Whether using mapping systems or conventional RF ablation techniques, clinicians still rely on X-ray images to position and guide catheters. Thus, exploiting X-ray image information is crucial for providing additional information to clinicians during cardiac ablation procedures.

Hence, there has been a trend lately of researchers investigating image-based solutions since these would also provide inexpensive and simple assistance to clinicians and could alleviate some of the burdens involved with the commercially available expensive technologies. We have identified three recent works that focus on the detection and tracking aspects of catheters visible in X-ray images [51-53].

These works address some of the inherent properties associated with the acquisition of X-ray images: (i) low quality and characterized by low signal to noise ratios, (ii) the non-rigid catheters visible in them have foreshortening artifacts due to X-ray projection principles, (iii) catheters may be occluded or overlapped by other catheters or background artifacts, and (iv) specifically during real-time fluoroscopic guidance, one can also observe motion blur artifacts.

i. Detection of catheters

The goal of any algorithm is to find all potential catheter electrode candidates in the X-ray images. The key is to perform these detections without the requirement of user interactivity or algorithm re-initialization. Once candidate electrodes are estimated these need to be subsequently filtered to remove false positives (outliers).

In current research practice, the 'blob detector' formulation is used to detect electrodes. We recall that electrodes appearances are not always the same in X-ray images due to foreshortening and projective effects. They can appear larger or smaller and their shape can change from rectangular → elliptical → circular over consecutive frames. It should be noted that for an individual X-ray image, the appearance of the electrodes belonging to the same catheter are very similar: if one of them appears as a circle it is very likely that the others share the same appearance. The candidate electrodes are obtained from a blobness measure influenced by non-maximum suppression. This blobness measure is implicitly greater than one since we are using a scale-space approach to detect electrodes at different scales. In other words, a catheter tip electrode will appear larger than the other electrodes.

Authors in [51, 53] investigated different methods that yield different performances both w.r.t. the detection rate and execution time. These approaches are based respectively on the usage of a "laplacian of gaussian" (LoG) and a "difference of gaussian" (DoG). The (LoG) blob detector [54] is a non-separable linear filter capable of finding blob-like structures while having low responses to edge-like structures. For each X-ray image it is necessary to run three linear filters and to evaluate the blobness measure:

$$Blobness_{LoG}(x, y, t_0) = t_0\left(L_{xx} L_{yy} - L_{xy}^2\right) \tag{1}$$

where L_{xx}, L_{yy}, L_{xy} are respectively the convolution of the X-ray image I(x,y) with G_{xx}, G_{yy}, G_{xy} being the second derivatives of the gaussian filter and $t_0 = \sigma^2$ is used for normalization purposes equal to the variance of the gaussian filter.

The (DoG) blob detector [55] is an approximation of the "laplacian of gaussian" filter and is based only on the usage of gaussian filters that are linearly separable. A scale-space representation of the image is obtained by filtering the image with a gaussian kernel using increasing variances. The difference between two neighboring scale-space images is taken and this latter result is used as a blobness measure. The mathematical formulation for the 2D gaussian filter is:

$$G(u, v, t_0) = \frac{1}{\sqrt{2\pi t_0}} e^{-(u^2 + v^2)/(2t_0)} \tag{2}$$

and the blobness measure becomes:

$$Blobness_{DoG}(x, y, t_0) = I(x, y) * G(x, y, kt_0) - I(x, y) * G(x, y, t_0) \tag{3}$$

This detector has a significant response in correspondence to edge-like features in the image and thus yields more outliers (i.e. higher false positives) when compared to the LoG detector. False positive candidate electrodes exist. To eliminate these, a Top-Hat filter is implemented which discards candidates that do not fulfill spatial and geometric constraint characteristics of an electrode. Since we are looking for "quasi circular" candidates mimicking electrodes, a structuring element with a circular diameter of 15 pixels is used. This immediately removes the majority of outliers. Second, since an electrode is metallic (and thus radiopaque), it appears as a very dark cluster in the X-ray image. Thus, candidate electrodes appearing as a bright cluster are rejected. From this, the blobness measure can be used to distinguish between catheter tips and other electrodes (tip-electrodes have a stronger measure as they are larger in size). For the sake of brevity, we direct readers to [51, 53] for additional details on the various outlier removal methods. Figure 4 and Figure 5 show intermediate and final results of image-based catheter detection solutions. The accuracy of the techniques is well above 95% when compared to ground-truth data.

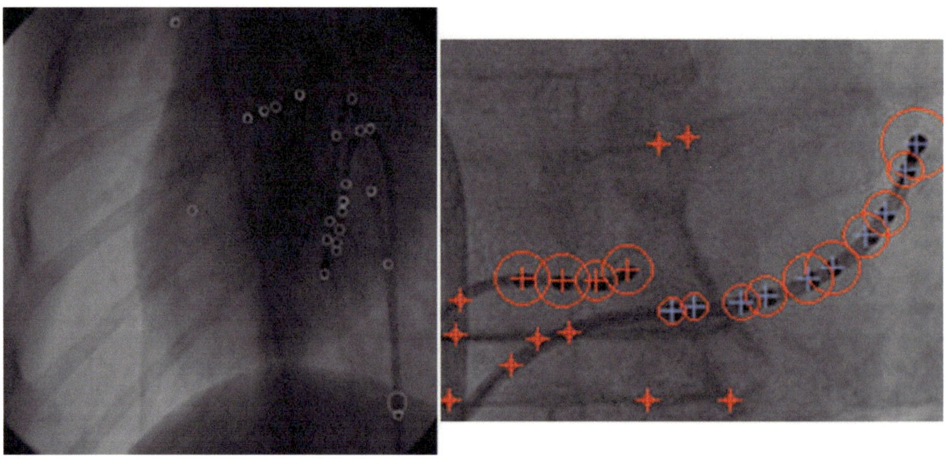

Figure 4. Examples of blob detections in X-ray images of dog (*left*) and patient (*right*). Images taken respectively from [51] and [53].

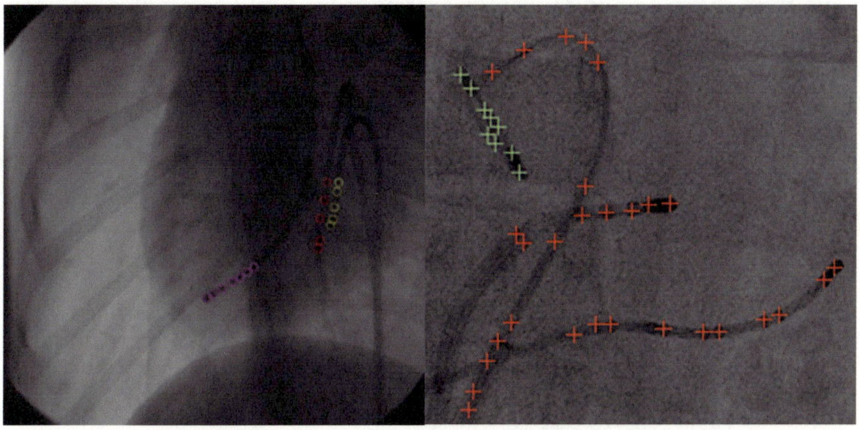

Figure 5. Example images of complete catheter detections in dog (*left*) and patient (*right*), after outlier removal. The different color coding implies detections of different catheter types. Images taken respectively from [51] and [53].

ii. Tracking of catheters

Initial solutions for tracking catheters in X-ray are presented in [52, 53]. In clinical practice, X-ray fluoroscopy images are acquired at about 15 frames per second depending on the system settings. Thus, developing image-based solutions that track at the rate of several images per second would be considered as an acceptable efficiency. The accuracy requirements depend on the specific application, and millimeter accuracy is roughly comparable with the currently available mapping navigation systems, while others [56, 57] have found 2-mm accuracy to be sufficient. Since the clinician needs to position the ablation catheter on heart tissue as it performs the burning, the most vital information to be tracked accurately is the catheter tip electrode. A very low false positive rate is also important to reduce any risk of inaccurate or insufficient treatment [52]. As seen in Figure 4-5, it is common practice that more than one catheter is used simultaneously; therefore, the ability to track multiple catheters is also an important requirement satisfied by image-based tracking solutions. For example, tracking the coronary sinus (CS) catheter can be used for transseptal puncture guidance [52, 58] and respiratory motion correction [52, 59]. There are several studies on the feasibility and significance of such a method for fluoroscopic-based guidance and mapping. Philips Healthcare has a product called the *EP navigator* that requires a user operator to indicate the position of the ablation catheter on the X-ray image ('point tagging'). It was evaluated during a catheter ablation [60], while the authors in [61] found it feasible to use their automatic catheter tracking method in a clinical environment.

In [52], authors introduce an efficient and robust method for multiple catheter detection and tracking. The proposed technique exploits the clinical setup knowledge to provide search constraints and boost both speed and accuracy. The method involves user input only in the beginning of the case, and runs fully automatically for the rest of the intervention. The method is based on a computationally efficient geodesic framework to trace the sheath and to find one or multiple catheter tips. The method was validated on 1107 fluoroscopic images taken from four patients from different clinics, demonstrating robust multiple catheters tracking at 10 images/s. The complete details of the algorithm are found in [52]. Figure 6 shows intermediate and final results of catheter detection.

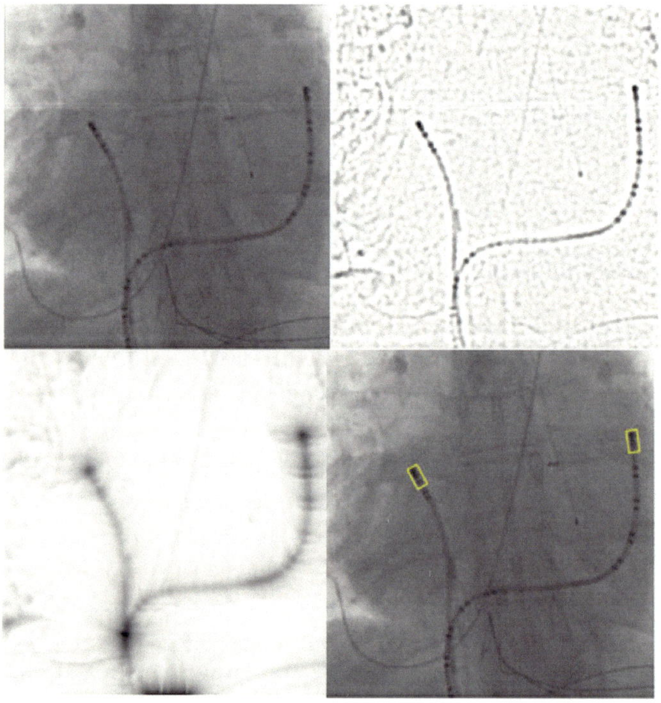

Figure 6. The original X-ray image with preprocessing (*top-row*) followed by geodesics properties computation. Final tip electrodes boxed in yellow (*bottom-row*).

Lastly, as an alternative tracking solution, authors in [53] develop a template-based approach. Tracking methods are initialized using the basic detection algorithm of LoG or DoG. This detection is used to create a customized 2D catheter model comprising a connected graph which gives information about the initial shape and orientation of the catheter. In subsequent X-ray image frames, the tracking methods use the same blob detection method and a modified catheter detection method that uses the customized model of the catheter being used during intervention [53]. Incorporating the customized model may allow successful tracking in cases where some catheter electrodes are overlapped with other dense objects or are outside the field of view. The current implementation requires manual detection of failed tracking, at which point the operator can restart with the basic detection algorithm [53].

iii. Future trends

There is room to investigate the above methods under various clinical conditions and different C-arm fluoroscopy devices. The variety in image quality in clinical cases is due to the variability in patient size, the variability in the image content with the presence of additional or implanted devices that were not used in our animal experiment. These must be accounted for when improving results [62]. Ultimately, achieving automatic detections and tracking can simplify 3D reconstruction of electrodes using single or multi-view approaches [63-64].

3. Conclusions

In summary, this chapter presented the latest findings involving the detection and tracking of cardiac ablation catheters. Several commercial 3D mapping systems provide non-fluoroscopic catheters with magnetic tips. These are detected and tracked in real-time using custom hardware and are used in everyday practice in luminary hospitals. Conventional RF ablation is still a requirement in many hospitals worldwide that cannot afford the expensive 3D mapping technologies. The advantages of image-based tracking technologies are many including being inexpensive and practical. With the advent of real-time computing capabilities, speed is a non-issue. However, researchers must continue to focus their efforts on developing mature algorithms for robust tracking – with the right catheter models. The keys for robustness against large data variation from fluoroscopic sequences involve considering machine learning approaches and obtaining large data sets for training and quantitative evaluation.

Acknowledgements

Dr. Pascal Fallavollita would like to acknowledge the support of the Chair for Computer Aided Medical Procedures & Augmented Reality, Technische Universität München.

Author details

Pascal Fallavollita*

Chair for Computer Aided Medical Procedures & Augmented Reality, Fakultät für Informatik, Technische Universität München, Germany

References

[1] Kumar; Abbas; Fausto. Robbins and Cotran Pathologic Basis of Disease (7th ed.). Philadelphia: Elsevier Saunders; 2005. p556.

[2] The Johns Hopkins Hospital, and Johns Hopkins Health System: http://www.hopkinsmedicine.org/healthlibrary/conditions/cardiovascular_diseases/anatomy_and_function_of_the_hearts_electrical_system_85,P00214/ (accessed November 18, 2013)

[3] Deo, Rajat, and Christine M. Albert. Epidemiology and genetics of sudden cardiac death. *Circulation* 2012; 125(4), 620-637.

[4] Lloyd-Jones D, Adams RJ, Brown TM, Carnethon M, Dai S, De Simone G, Ferguson TB, Ford E, Furie K, Gillespie C, Go A, Greenlund K, Haase N, Hailpern S, Ho PM, Howard V, Kissela B, Kittner S, Lackland D, Lisabeth L, Marelli A, McDermott MM, Meigs J, Mozaffarian D, Mussolino M, Nichol G, Roger VL, Rosamond W, Sacco R, Sorlie P, Thom T, Wasserthiel-Smoller S, Wong ND, Wylie-Rosett J. Heart disease and stroke statistics–2010 update: a report from the American Heart Association. *Circulation* 2010; 121, e46-e215.

[5] Kong MH, Fonarow GC, Peterson ED, Curtis AB, Hernandez AF, Sanders GD, Thomas KL, Hayes DL, Al-Khatib SM. Systematic review of the incidence of sudden cardiac death in the United States. *J Am Coll Cardiol* 2011; 57, 794-801.

[6] Nichol G, Thomas E, Callaway CW, Hedges J, Powell JL, Aufderheide TP, Rea T, Lowe R, Brown T, Dreyer J, Davis D, Idris A, Stiell I. Regional variation in out-of-hospital cardiac arrest incidence and outcome. *JAMA* 2008; 300, 1423-1431.

[7] Chugh SS, Jui J, Gunson K, Stecker EC, John BT, Thompson B, Ilias N, Vickers C, Dogra V, Daya M, Kron J, Zheng ZJ, Mensah G, McAnulty J. Current burden of sudden cardiac death: multiple source surveillance versus retrospective death certificate-based review in a large U.S. Community. *J Am Coll Cardiol* 2004; 44, 1268-1275.

[8] de Vreede-Swagemakers JJ, Gorgels AP, Dubois-Arbouw WI, van Ree JW, Daemen MJ, Houben LG, Wellens HJ. Out-of-hospital cardiac arrest in the 1990's: a population-based study in the Maastricht area on incidence, characteristics and survival. *J Am Coll Cardiol* 1997; 30, 1500-1505.

[9] Byrne R, Constant O, Smyth Y, Callagy G, Nash P, Daly K, Crowley J. Multiple source surveillance incidence and aetiology of out-of-hospital sudden cardiac death in a rural population in the west of Ireland. *Eur Heart J* 2008; 29, 1418-1423.

[10] Hua W, Zhang LF, Wu YF, Liu XQ, Guo DS, Zhou HL, Gou ZP, Zhao LC, Niu HX, Chen KP, Mai JZ, Chu LN, Zhang S. Incidence of sudden cardiac death in China: analysis of 4 regional populations. *J Am Coll Cardiol* 2009; 54, 1110-1118.

[11] Ford ES, Ajani UA, Croft JB, Critchley JA, Labarthe DR, Kottke TE, Giles WH, Capewell S. Explaining the decrease in U.S. Deaths from coronary disease, 1980–2000. *N Engl J Med* 2007; 356, 2388-2398.

[12] Rosamond WD, Chambless LE, Folsom AR, Cooper LS, Conwill DE, Clegg L, Wang CH, Heiss G. Trends in the incidence of myocardial infarction and in mortality due to coronary heart disease, 1987 to 1994. *N Engl J Med* 1998; 339, 861-867.

[13] Fox CS, Evans JC, Larson MG, Kannel WB, Levy D. Temporal trends in coronary heart disease mortality and sudden cardiac death from 1950 to 1999: the Framingham Heart Study. *Circulation* 2004; 110, 522-527.

[14] Zheng ZJ, Croft JB, Giles WH, Mensah GA. Sudden cardiac death in the United States, 1989 to 1998. *Circulation* 2001; 104, 2158-2163.

[15] Dudas K, Lappas G, Stewart S, Rosengren A. Trends in out-of-hospital deaths due to coronary heart disease in Sweden (1991 to 2006). *Circulation* 2011; 123, 46-52.

[16] Gerber Y, Jacobsen SJ, Frye RL, Weston SA, Killian JM, Roger VL. Secular trends in deaths from cardiovascular diseases: a 25-year community study. *Circulation* 2006; 113, 2285-2292.

[17] Myerburg RJ, Interian A, Simmons J, Castellanos A. Sudden cardiac death. In: Zipes DP, ed. Cardiac Electrophysiology: From Cell to Bedside. Philadelphia, PA: WB Saunders; 2004; 720-731.

[18] Cobb LA, Fahrenbruch CE, Olsufka M, Copass MK. Changing incidence of out-of-hospital ventricular fibrillation, 1980–2000. *JAMA* 2002; 288, 3008-3013.

[19] Joseph, J. P., and K. Rajappan. "Radiofrequency ablation of cardiac arrhythmias: past, present and future." *QJM* 2012; 105(4), 303-314.

[20] Scheinman MM, Morady F, Hess DS, Gonzalez R. Catheter-induced ablation of the atrioventricular junction to control refractory supraventricular arrhythmias. *JAMA* 1982; 248, 851.

[21] Gallagher JJ, Svenson RH, Kasell JH, German LD, Bardy GH, Broughton A, et al. Catheter technique for closed-chest ablation of the atrioventricular conduction system. *N Engl J Med* 1982; 306, 194.

[22] Weber H, Schmitz L. Catheter technique for closed-chest ablation of an accessory atrioventricular pathway. *N Engl J Med* 1983; 308, 653.

[23] Morady F, Scheinman MM. Transvenous catheter ablation of a posteroseptal accessory pathway in a patient with the Wolff-Parkinson-White syndrome. *N Engl J Med* 1984; 310, 705.

[24] Haissaguerre M, Warin JF, Lemetayer P, Saoudi N, Guillem JP, Blanchot P. Closed-chest ablation of retrograde conduction in patients with atrioventricular nodal reentrant tachycardia. *N Engl J Med* 1989; 320, 426.

[25] Hartzler GO. Electrode catheter ablation of refractory focal ventricular tachycardia. *J Am Coll Cardiol* 1983; 2, 1107.

[26] Jackman WM, Wang X, Friday KJ, Roman CA, Moulton KP, Beckman KJ, et al. Catheter ablation of accessory atrioventricular pathways by radiofrequency current. *N Engl J Med* 1991; 324,1605.

[27] Calkins H, Sousa J, El-Atassi R, Rosenheck S, de Buitleir M, Kou WH, et al. Diagnosis and cure of the Wolff-Parkinson-White syndrome of paroxysmal supraventricular tachycardia during a single electrophysiologic test. *N Engl J Med* 1991; 324, 1612.

[28] Huang SK, Bharati S, Graham AR, Lev M, Marcus FI, Odell RC, et al. Closed chest catheter dessication of the atrioventricular junction using radiofrequency energy — a new method of catheter ablation. *J Am Coll Cardiol* 1987; 9, 349.

[29] Kay GN, Epstein AE, Dailey SM, Plumb VJ. Role of radiofrequency ablation in the management of supraventricular arrhythmias: Experience in 760 consecutive patients. *J Cardiovasc Electrophysiol* 1993; 4, 371.

[30] Nath S, DiMarco JP, Haines DE. Basic aspects of radiofrequency ablation. *J Cardiovasc Electrophysiol* 1994; 5, 863.

[31] Dinerman JL, Berger RD, Calkins H. Temperature monitoring during radiofrequency ablation. *J Cardiovasc Electrophysiol* 1996; 7, 163.

[32] Jais P, Shah DC, Haissaguerre M, Hocini M, Garrigue S, Le Metayer P, et al. Prospective randomized comparison of irrigated-tip versus conventional-tip catheters for ablation of common flutter. *Circulation* 2000; 101, 772.

[33] Ruffy R, Imran MA, Santel DJ, Wharton JM. Radiofrequency delivery through a cooled catheter tip allows the creation of larger endomyocardial lesions in the ovine heart. *J Cardiovasc Electrophysiol* 1995; 6, 1089.

[34] Yamane T, Jais P, Shah DC, Hocini M, Peng JT, Deisenhofer I, et al. Efficacy and safety of an irrigated-tip catheter for the ablation of accessory pathways resistant to conventional radiofrequency ablation. *Circulation* 2000; 102, 2565.

[35] Soejima K, Delacretaz E, Suzuki M, Brunckhorst CB, Maisel WH, Friedman PL, et al. Saline-cooled versus standard radiofrequency catheter ablation for infarct-related ventricular tachycardias. *Circulation* 2001; 103, 1858.

[36] Boston Scientific website. http://www.bostonscientific.com/us/ep.html. (accessed November 18, 2013)

[37] Biosense Webster Website. http://www.biosensewebster.com/ (accessed November 18, 2013)

[38] Calkins, Hugh, et al. "2012 HRS/EHRA/ECAS Expert Consensus Statement on Catheter and Surgical Ablation of Atrial Fibrillation: Recommendations for Patient Selection, Procedural Techniques, Patient Management and Follow-up, Definitions, Endpoints, and Research Trial Design A report of the Heart Rhythm Society (HRS) Task Force on Catheter and Surgical Ablation of Atrial Fibrillation. Developed in partnership with the European Heart Rhythm Association (EHRA), a registered branch of the European Society of Cardiology (ESC) and...." Europace 2012; 14(4), 528-606.

[39] Camm AJ, Kirchhof P, Lip GY, et al. Guidelines for the management of atrial fibrillation: the Task Force for the Management of Atrial Fibrillation of the European Society of Cardiology (ESC). *Eur Heart J* 2010; 31(19), 2369 -2429.

[40] Perisinakis K, Damilakis J, Theocharopoulos N, Manios E, Vardas P, Gourtsoyiannis N. Accurate assessment of patient effective radiation dose and associated detriment risk from radiofrequency catheter ablation procedures. Circulation 2001; 104(1), 58-62.

[41] Steven D, Servatius H, Rostock T, et al. Reduced fluoroscopy during atrial fibrillation ablation: benefits of robotic guided navigation. *J Cardiovasc Electrophysiol* 2010; 21(1), 6-12.

[42] Pascal Fallavollita. The Future of Cardiac Mapping, *Cardiac Arrhythmias- New Considerations*, Prof. Francisco R. Breijo-Marquez (Ed.), InTech; 2012.

[43] Andrew D'Silva and Matthew Wright, Advances in Imaging for Atrial Fibrillation Ablation. *Radiology Research and Practice* 2011; vol. 2011..

[44] Casella, M., Pelargonio, G., Russo, A. D., Riva, S., Bartoletti, S., Santangeli, P.,... & Tondo, C. Near-zero fluoroscopic exposure in supraventricular arrhythmia ablation using the EnSite NavX™ mapping system: personal experience and review of the literature. *Journal of interventional cardiac electrophysiology* 2011; 31(2), 109-118.

[45] LaPage, Martin Ja; Saul, J Philipb. Update on rhythm mapping and catheter navigation. *Current Opinion in Cardiology* 2011, 26(2), 79–85.

[46] Yamada T, Doppalapudi H, McElderry HT, et al.: Idiopathic ventricular arrhythmias originating from the papillary muscles in the left ventricle: prevalence, electrocardiographic and electrophysiological characteristics, and results of the radiofrequency catheter ablation. *J Cardiovasc Electrophysiol* 2010; 21, 62–69.

[47] Georg Nölker, Klaus-Jürgen Gutleben, Stefan Asbach, Jürgen Vogt, Johannes Heintze, Johannes Brachmann, et al. Intracardiac echocardiography for registration of rotational angiography-based left atrial reconstructions: a novel approach integrating two intraprocedural three-dimensional imaging techniques in atrial fibrillation ablation. *Europace* 2011; 13 (4), 492-498.

[48] LaPage, Martin Ja; Saul, J Philipb. Update on rhythm mapping and catheter navigation. *Current Opinion in Cardiology* 2011; 26(2), 79–85.

[49] M. Azizian and R. Patel. Intraoperative 3D stereo visualization for image-guided cardiac ablation. *SPIE Medical Imaging: Visualization, Image-Guided Procedures, and Modeling*, 2011; 7964, 79640F.

[50] Winkle, Roger A., et al. Physician-controlled costs: the choice of equipment used for atrial fibrillation ablation. *Journal of Interventional Cardiac Electrophysiology* 2013; 1-9.

[51] Milletari, Fausto, Nassir Navab, and Pascal Fallavollita. Automatic Detection of Multiple and Overlapping EP Catheters in Fluoroscopic Sequences. *Medical Image Com-*

puting and Computer-Assisted Intervention–MICCAI. Springer Berlin Heidelberg, 2013; 371-379.

[52] Yatziv, L., Chartouni, M., Datta, S., & Sapiro, G. Toward multiple catheters detection in fluoroscopic image guided interventions. *Information Technology in Biomedicine, IEEE Transactions on* 2012; 16(4), 770-781.

[53] Ma, YingLiang, et al. Real-time x-ray fluoroscopy-based catheter detection and tracking for cardiac electrophysiology interventions. *Medical Physics* 2013; 40(7), 071902.

[54] T. Lindeberg.: Detecting salient blob-like image structures and their scales with a scale-space primal sketch: a method for focus-of-attention. *IJCV* 1993; 11(3), 283-318.

[55] Lowe, David G., Chris Murphy.: Distinctive Image Features from Scale-Invariant Key-points. IJCV 2004; 60(2), 91-110.

[56] D. R. Elgort, E. Y. Wong, C. M. Hillenbrand, F. K. Wacker, J. S. Lewin, and J. L. Duerk, Real-time catheter tracking and adaptive imaging. *J. Magn. Reson. Imag* 2003; 18(5), 621-626..

[57] S. A. M. Baert, M. A. Viergever, and W. J. Niessen, Guide wire tracking during endovascular interventions. *IEEE Trans. Med. Imag*. 2003; 22(8), 965-972.

[58] F. Bourier, A. Brost, L. Yatziv, J. Hornegger, N. Strobel, and K. Kurzidim. (2010). Coronary sinus extraction for multimodality registration to guide transseptal puncture, in Proc. 8th Intervent. MRI Symp., pp. 311–313. [Online]. Available: http:// www5.informatik.unierlangen. de/Forschung/Publikationen/2010/Bou rier10-CSE.pdf

[59] Ma, Ying Liang, et al. Real-time respiratory motion correction for cardiac electrophysiology procedures using image-based coronary sinus catheter tracking. *Medical Image Computing and Computer-Assisted Intervention–MICCAI*. Springer Berlin Heidelberg, 2010; 391-399.

[60] Knecht, S., Skali, H., O'neill, M. D., Wright, M., Matsuo, S., Chaudhry, G. M.,... & Jaïs, P. Computed tomography–fluoroscopy overlay evaluation during catheter ablation of left atrial arrhythmia. *Europace* 2008; 10(8), 931-938.

[61] De Buck, Stijn, et al. Toward image-based catheter tip tracking for treatment of atrial fibrillation. *CI2BM09-MICCAI Workshop on Cardiovascular Interventional Imaging and Biophysical Modelling* 2009.

[62] Heibel H, Glocker B, Groher M, Pfister M, Navab N.: Interventional tool tracking using discrete optimization. *IEEE Trans Med Imaging* 2013; 32(3), 544-55.

[63] Pascal Fallavollita.: Is Single-View Fluoroscopy Sufficient in Guiding Cardiac Ablation Procedures? *International Journal of Biomedical Imaging* 2010; vol. 2010, 13 pages.

[64] Pascal Fallavollita.: Acquiring Multiview C-Arm Images to Assist Cardiac Ablation Procedures. *European Association for Signal Processing: Journal on Image and Video Processing* 2010; vol. 2010, 10 pages.

Chapter 4

Ventricular Arrhythmia Risk in Noncardiac Diseases

Ioana Mozos

Additional information is available at the end of the chapter

http://dx.doi.org/10.5772/57164

1. Introduction

Electrocardiographic changes were mentioned in several noncardiac diseases, due to multiple mechanisms: changes of the position of the heart, autonomic imbalance, hormonal abnormalities, interposition of fluid or tissue between the heart and the electrodes, increased blood pressure, cardiomyopathy of systemic diseases, electrolyte imbalances, or due to therapy [1, 2].

A prolonged ECG *QT interval* and an increased *QT dispersion* (QTd, the difference between the longest and shortest QT interval duration in all 12 standard ECG leads), are markers of ventricular arrythmia risk. Sudden cardiac death, a major public health problem, is caused, mainly, by ventricular fibrillation [3].

Besides a prolonged QT interval, longer than 450 ms in male and 460 ms in female [4], *late ventricular potentials* (LVPs), which are low amplitude and high frequency waveforms, appearing in the terminal part of the QRS complex, and are markers of an electrophysiological substrate for reentry ventricular arrythmias in a diseased myocardium, were also detected in several extracardiac diseases using signal averaged ECG [5].

Standard 12-lead ECG provides a bedside snapshot of the electrial activity of the heart, but *Holter electrocardiogarphy* enables detection of episodes of arrhythmia and evaluate therapeutic interventions [6].

2. Objective

The aim of the present chapter was to provide a concise overview of available data regarding epidemiology and pathophysiology of ventricular arrhythmias in several noncardiac

INTECH
open science | open minds

© 2014 Mozos; licensee InTech. This is a paper distributed under the terms of the Creative Commons Attribution License (http://creativecommons.org/licenses/by/3.0), which permits unrestricted use, distribution, and reproduction in any medium, provided the original work is properly cited.

diseases, to mention the main methods used to assess arrhythmia risk, as well as to elucidate their relation to long-term outcome. Dyslipidemia, obesity, diabetes mellitus, liver, hematologic, neurologic and psychiatric disorders, are discussed.

3. Dyslipidaemia and ventricular arrhythmia risk

Elevated LDL cholesterol was associated with all manifestations of coronary artery disease including sudden cardiac death [7]. *Hypercholesterolemia* is not only atherogenic, but is also associated with autonomic imbalance, alteration of the contractile properties of the myocardium, increased oxidative stress and ventricular electrophysiological remodeling [8, 9]. Myocardial electrical remodeling due to hypercholesterolemia caused prolonged action potential durations, longer QTc (heart rate corrected QT interval durations), conduction slowing and increased repolarization dispersion [9, 10].

Several clinical and autopsy studies demonstrated an association between elevated cholesterol levels and sudden cardiac death [11, 12]. Gualdiero et al. reported a positive correlation between cholesterol level, QT dispersion and premature ventricular contractions in patients with isolated hypercholesterolemia, and normalization of serum cholesterol and QT dispersion and improvement of ventricular ectopic activity, with simvastatin [13]. Szabo et al. found significant correlations of QT interval duration and QT dispersion with total and LDL cholesterol, triglycerides and apoplipoprotein B, respectively, in patients with *type IIb hyperlipoproteinemia*, without myocardial ischemia, suggesting a direct effect of hyperlipidemia on ventricular repolarization [14]. LDL increases the cholesterol to phospholipid ratio in the cell membrane, enhancing membrane rigidity and impairing functionality of the ion channels and ventricular repolarization [14, 15]. Ventricular repolarization is reflected by the QT interval on the ECG, which is regulated mainly by potassium channels. On the other hand, type II hyperlipoproteinemia is characterized by accelerated atherosclerosis, related to small dense LDL synthesis.

It was also hypothesized that hypercholesterolemia causes repolarization abnormalities, probably, by beta or IK channel phosphorylation mediated mechanisms [9]. Hypercholesterolemia causes also endothelial dysfunction, with impaired microvascular vasodilatation, facilitating vasoconstriction, and electrical heterogeneity and extrasystolic activity [13]. The increase in the QT interval duration in cholesterol fed rabbits was lesser if L-Arginine was supplemented, suggesting a beneficial role of L-Arginine (a nitric acid precusror) in hypercholesterolemia induced repolarization characteristics [9]. L-Arginine increases endogenous nitric oxide, which may activate ATP dependent K channels, shortening the action potential [9].

Late ventricular potentials were detected in patients with high and moderately elevated serum cholesterol [5, 16].

Statins have antiarrhythmic properties, exhibiting a protective effect against the occurrence of ventricular arrhythmias and atrial fibrillation, in addition to their lipid-lowering and anti-atherogenic effects [5, 12, 13, 17, 18]. The main mechanisms explaining, probably, the antiarrhythmic properties of statins are as follows: prevention of ischemia-induced electrophysiological effects that predispose to ventricular arrhythmias and ischemia-induced oxidative stress, decrease in ischemia-induced myocyte hypertrophy, reverse of neural remodeling induced by hypercholesterolemia, increase of heart rate variability, decrease of QT interval duration and variability, reversion of electrophysiological remodeling induced by hypercholesterolemia, increase in parasympathetic tone, changes in transmembrane ion channel properties, decrease of the incidence of late ventricular potentials [10, 12].

4. Ventricular arrhythmias in obesity and eating disorders

Morbid *obesity* was associated with high rates of sudden cardiac death [19, 20]. Lalani et al. reported a high prevalence of abnormal signal averaged ECGs in obese without known cardiovascular disease [20]. An increased QT dispersion was found in obese women, associated with left ventricular hypertrophy [21] and prolonged QT intervals were measured in obese patients [22-24]. Several mechanisms explain the high sudden cardiac death risk in obese, including: parasympathetic withdrawal, conduction abnormalities, cardiomyopathy of obesity with cardiomegaly and myocyte hypertrohy, lipotoxicity of the myocardium induced by free fatty acids, released from hypertrophied adipocytes in obese persons with myocardial steatosis, structural heterogeneity due to fatty infiltration of the heart, focal myocardial disarray, fibrosis and mononuclear cell infiltration [5, 19, 20, 25, 26]. Premature ventricular contractions (PVCs) are very prevalent in obese [27] and sudden cardiac death risk is increased in obese compared to normal weighted survivors of a myocardial infarction [28].

Weight loss causes a shortening of the QT interval, correlated with diastolic blood pressure decrease, and changes in time and frequency domain parameters of heart rate variability, with recovery of the physiological autonomic control (increase in parasympathetic and reduction in sympathetic indices [29].

QT prolongation, signal averaged ECG abnormalities and late ventricular potentials were reported in *eating disorders*, including both anorexia and bulimia nervosa [30]. Bulimia nervosa, an eating disorder characterized by binge eating and purging, was associated with QT interval prolongation, related to electrolyte imbalances, especially hypokalemia [31]. Anorexia nervosa carries the highest mortality of any psychiatric disorder, very often attributable to sudden cardiac death. Delayed cardiac repolarization and QT prolongation, not correlated with disease severity, were reported [32]. Any patient with an eating disorder should undergo standard 12-lead ECG.

Disease	Mechanisms	Methods and arrhythmia
Obesity	parasympathetic withdrawal, conduction abnormalities, cardiomyopathy of obesity, lipotoxicity of the myocardium induced by free fatty acids, structural heterogeneity due to fatty infiltration of the heart, focal myocardial disarray, fibrosis, mononuclear cell infiltration	SAECG QTd QT PVCs
Hypercholesterolemia	autonomic imbalance, endothelial dysfunction, oxidative stress, impaired functionality of ion channels	QTc QTd LVPs PVCs
Anorexia nervosa, Bulimia nervosa	electrolyte imbalances (hypokalemia)	QT, LVPs
Diabetes mellitus	autonomic imbalance, oxidative stress, increased cytosolic calcium, increased Na current, hyperinsulinemia, insulinresitance, hypokalemia	QT, QTd LVPs
Liver cirrhosis	cirrhotic cardiomyopathy, cardiac ion channel remodeling, electrolyte imbalances, impaired autonomic function	QT
Stroke, Subarachnoid hemorrhage	cardiac autonomic imbalance, neural interventions, norepinephrine, calcium influx, myocytolysis, hypokalemia, concomitant myocardial ischemia and heart failure, risk factors for coronary heart disease, aging, inflammation, Takotsubo cardiomyopathy	QT QTd VT, R/T, VF, Vf Holter monitoring
Intracranial hemorrhage	intraventricular blood, hydrocephalus	QTc PVCs, TdP
Neuromuscular disorders	cardiomyopathy, diffuse cardiac fibrosis and fatty acid infiltration, myocyte degeneration	QTcd, JTcd QTc, LVPs
Parkinson's disease	autonomic disturbance (intrinsic or iatrogenic), cardiovascular comorbidities, electrolyte imbalances, degeneration of cardioselective neurons	QT
Epilepsy	sympathovagal imbalance, impaired cardiac repolarization, dysfunction of cortical networks, ictal hypoxemia and hypercapnia, stress hormones, cardiorespiratory interactions, fibrosis (perivascular, interstitial)	QT QTd LVPs PVCs
Anemia	left ventricular hypertrophy, sympathetic nervous system activation, oxidative stress, chronic inflammation, decreased myocardial oxygen supply	QT QTd LVPs

Table 1. Mechanisms of ventricular arrhythmias and methods used to assess sudden cardiac risk in some extracardiac diseases

http://dx.doi.org/10.5772/57164

5. Glucose metabolism disorders and ventricular arrhythmia risk

Several studies associate diabetes mellitus and hyperglycemia with sudden cardiac death, related to QT interval prolongation, appearance of late ventricular potentials, impaired depolarization and repolarization, enhanced sympathetic activity, oxidative stress, increased cytosolic calcium content, defective phosphoinositide 3-kinase signaling with increased persistent sodium current, premature and accelerated atherosclerosis, transient hypoglycemic episodes due to drug therapy, duration of diabetes, and renal failure, as target-organ damage, causing electrolyte imbalances [5, 33-36]. QT interval prolongation and increase of QT dispersion are predictive for sudden cardiac death in patients with *type 1 and 2 diabetes mellitus* [37]. QT interval duration was independently associated with glycated hemoglobin in patients with type 1 diabetes mellitus [38], and hyperinsulinemia and insulinresistance can contribute to QTc prolongation [39]. Li et al found a high prevalence of prolonged QTc intervals, and low height, high waist circumference, increased diastolic blood pressure levels, high postprandial glucose levels, high fasting insulin and presence of microalbuminuria, as risk factors for QTc prolongation among Chinese patients with type 2 diabetes mellitus [40].

Stress hyperglycemia on admission was found to be a predictor of mortality and arrhythmias in patients with acute myocardial infarction and could be used in the stratification of risk in these patients [5, 41, 42]. An independent association between hyperglycemia and prolonged QTc and increased QT dispersion was found in healthy, nondiabetic subjects [39].

Severe *hypoglycemia* is also associated with ventricular repolarization abnormalities, prolongation of the QT interval, and ventricular arrhythmias [35]. QTc interval prolongation was observed during the episodes of sever hypoglycemia compared to the recovered stage, in patients with type 2 diabetes mellitus, associated with increase in serum catecholamines, altered neural regulation and hypokalemia [43, 44]. The likelihood of ventricular arrhythmias is increased, particularly when hypoglycemia occurs in a patient with autonomic neuropathy [35]. Sudden nocturnal death in young people with type 1 diabetes could be due to cardiac arrhythmias induced by hypoglycemia [45]. Hypokalemia, caused by hyperinsulinemia and intracellular shift of potassium, could explain the altered cardiac repolarization during the episodes of hypoglycemia [43].

6. Liver diseases and ventricular arrhythmia risk

Several cardiac problems have been reported in patienst with *liver cirrhosis,* including chronotrope incompetence, cardiomyopathy and prolonged QT intervals, proportional to the Child-Pugh class [46]. A prolonged QT interval represents the most common electrocardiographic (ECG) finding in patients with liver cirrhosis and is the electrophysiological hallmark of "cirrhotic cardiomyopathy" [47, 48, 49]. Cirrhotic cardiomyopathy can appear in all forms of cirrhosis and includes systolic and diastolic dysfunction and electrophysiological abnormalities, in the absence of any known cardiac disease [48]. Cardiac ion channels remodeling has been noticed in patients with liver cirrhosis, with impaired K and Ca channels, due to endotoxins and increased biliary acids, which alter beta-adrenoreceptor, G protein and ionic channels in patients with cholestasis [46].

QT prolongation in liver pathology was first described in alcoholic liver diseases [50]. Alcohol effects on life-threatening arrhythmias correlate directly with the amount and duration of alcohol intake; even small quantities are significant in susceptible individuals [35]. Further studies reported prolonged QT intervals in patients with *primary biliary cirrhosis* and other *chronic non-alcoholic liver diseases,* related to the severity of the autonomic neuropathy, and could detect patients with increased cardiovascular risk [51]. QT interval prolongation was related to the pathophysiology of cirrhosis itself and not to a specific cause of cirrhosis [52]. Prolonged QTc intervals were related to the presence of portal hypertension, including mild portal hypertension, and liver dysfunction [53]. Genovesi et al. reported significant correlations between QTc and each of the following: plasma calcium level, portal hypertension, and the hepatic venous pressure gradient [47]. Liver disease severity, alcoholic etiology, and serum uric acid were associated with prolonged QT interval in patients with liver cirrhosis, according to another study [48]. *Liver transplantation* may revert cardiac dysfunction [54] and prolonged QTc returns to normal values, in most of the patients, after liver transplantation, suggesting that liver disease may not be the only factor in the pathogenesis of prolonged QTc [52, 55]. Acute gastrointestinal bleeding was found to further prolong QTc in patients with liver cirrhosis, and QTc prolongation predicted bleeding induced mortality [56].

Concluding, the mechanisms by which liver cirrhosis affects ventricular repolarization are as follows: electrolyte imbalances, impaired autonomic function, subclinical cardiomyopathy, reduced β-adrenoreceptor function, postreceptor pathway defects, altered physical properties of myocyte plasma membrane, elevated levels of cardiotoxins, ion channel remodeling, portosystemic shunting and systemic circulatory disturbances [46-48, 53, 54, 57].

The clinical significance of QT prolongation in liver cirrhosis is unclear, considering that sudden cardiac death and torsades de pointes are rare [58].

QTc interval was also measured in patients with *chronic hepatitis C,* showing non-significant increases six months after starting combination therapy with pegylated interferon and ribavirin, in order to achieve sustained virological response [59].

7. Cerebrogenic arrhythmias and ventricular arrhythmia risk in neurologic diseases

Cardiac diseases are a well-known *stroke* risk factors and complicate stroke outcome [60]. Cardiac arrhythmias and electrocardiographic abnormalities are frequently observed after acute cerebrovascular events, even in the absence of structural heart disease [61]. With improved survival after major cardiovascular events and aging of the population, stroke followed by myocardial infarction and arrhythmias will be an increasing clinical entity in the coming decades [60]. The neurologic event is the main cause of death only in the first week after stroke [62]. After the first year, cardiovascular diseases are the main cause of death in stroke patients [63]. Atrial fibrillation, the most common arrhythmia in clinical practice, is a major risk factor for embolic stroke [60, 64]. Stroke and *subarachnoid hemorrhage* cause other cerebrogenic ECG findings as well, prolong the QT interval, increase QT dispersion and ventricular arrhythmia risk, mainly due to an autonomic nervous system dysregulation [1, 61, 65, 66]. Large, inverted T waves following a prolonged QTc interval, common after subarachnoid hemorrhage, are often termed as "cerebral" or "neurogenic" [67]. Brady- and tachyarrhythmia, including polymorphic ventricular tachycardia (PVT), have been also described in the setting of neurologic injury [68]. The greatest risk of arrhythmias is, probably, within the first 24 h after stroke, with a marked decline in time [69]. Activation of both sympathetic and parasympathetic systems has cumulative effect in the development of arrhythmias and myocardial damage after cerebral incidents, and the damage of the hypothalamic, insular, and brainstem region is crucial for the genesis of cardiac arrhythmias, due to neural connections with other cortical sites and the autonomic nervous system [61]. Sander et al, found increased norepinephrine levels in patients with insular infarction, significantly related to adverse outcome and QTc [70]. The sympathetic system has a major role in the pathogenesis of hypokalemia and may indirectly result in QTc prolongation after subarachnoid hemorrhage [61]. Probably constant catecholamine stimulation of beta-adrenoreceptors linked to membrane Na^+/K^+-ATPases causes a potassium influx, resulting in hypokalemia, and thus precipitating ventricular arrhythmias [62]. Both reduced heart-rate variability (HRV) and impaired baroreceptor reflex sensitivity (BRS) suggest impaired physiological central and cardiac autonomic reflex function [62]. Ventricular arrhythmogenesis following stroke, related to the cardiac autonomic imbalance is explained by two hypotheses [62]. The first involves damage to central nervous structures controlling the autonomic nervous system, resulting in sympathetic amplification or parasympathetic inhibition, with subsequent ECG changes, without permanent myocardium damage, and the second hypothesis proposes an augmented sympathetic discharge, resulting in increased secretion of catecholamine, causing myocytolysis [62]. The insula plays an important role in autonomic nervous function imbalance after stroke [62, 71]. Involvement of the right insula decreases basal sympathetic tone and may result in parasympathetic hyperactivity, and left insular lesions decrease parasympathetic activity and augment cardiac sympathetic tone [71]. Sympathetic hyperactivity prolongs repolarization duration and increases arrhythmogenesis [62].

A concomitant myocardial ischemia or necrosis, elevated blood pressure and heart failure may be also considered [1]. Autopsy of stroke patients, who developed repolarization abnormalities, revealed no obvious coronary artery atherosclerosis in most of them, and the only findings were petechial subendocardial hemorrhages and focal myofibrillar degeneration, reproducible with intravenous administration of catecholamines or electrical stimulation of the vagus nerve in laboratory animals [61]. Sudden calcium influx, mediated by catecholamines, impairs myocardial relaxation, leads to myocytolysis, myofibrillar degeneration, coronary vasoconstriction, myocardial ischemia and ECG changes, and is proarrhythmic [61, 62]. Elevated serum uric acid, direct neural interventions, inflammation, reactive oxygen species, electrolyte imbalances, the structural and electrophysiological changes of a senescent heart and comorbities can increase sudden cardiac death risk in stroke [61, 66]. Stroke survivors with a prolonged QT in V6, were identified to have an increased sudden cardiac death risk [72]. Prolonged QT intervals were associated with decreased survival rates and worse neurological outcomes at hospital discharge [73]. The prevalence of cardiac arrhythmias after acute stroke may reach 28%, higher after subarachnoid hemorrhage (37.5%) and in right sided lesions [61]. The most prevalent ECG findings were, besides atrial fibrillation, sinus tachycardia, atrio-ventricular block, repolarization changes, premature ventricular contractions, R on T phenomenon (R/T), non-sustained, sustained and polymorphic ventricular tachycardia (VT), ventricular fibrillation (VF) and flutter (Vf) [61, 62]. Independent risk factors for the development of ventricular arrhythmias in patients with aneurysmal subarachnoid hemorrhage were prolonged QTc and decreased heart rate, and therapy with angiotensin converting enzyme inhibitors and angiotensin receptor blockers was protective [74]. Literature data are insufficient to support the hypothesis that subarachnoid hemorrhage and stroke cause ventricular arrhythmias, considering that in most patients additional QT prolonging causes were mentioned, including hypokalemia, hypomagnesaemia, and congenital long QT syndrome, and patients with stroke usually have risk factors for coronary artery disease, such as hypertension, diabetes mellitus, and smoking, or advanced age, or left ventricular hypertrophy [61, 62, 75]. Several studies did not control pre-existing arrhythmias, were of short duration and did not explore the long-term consequences of ventricular arrhythmogenesis [62]. Another important limitation of most of the studies is the use of single surface ECG, because it may underestimate arrhythmia incidence in the acute phase of a stroke [62]. Holter monitoring revealed a higher incidence of ventricular arrhythmias after transient ischemic attacks, cerebral infarction and intracerebral hemorrhage compared to patients who were not continuously monitored (56% vs. 8%) [76].

It is also possible that in some cases, prolonged QTc actually existed before the development of stroke and it could be used as a *predictor of future stroke* in the general population [75]. The association of QTc with cardiovascular risk factors does not fully explain the prognostic significance of QTc as a stroke predictor, but it is possible, that prolonged QTc interval is a marker of silent undetected atherosclerotic vascular disease [75]. QTc was previously associated with markers of subclinical atherosclerosis, including carotid intima media thickness, arterial stiffness and endothelial dysfunction [77-80]. Probably, QTc prolongation may be a surrogate indicator of subclinical atherosclerosis and subsequently can be predictive of future atherosclerotic vascular events such as stroke, but it is not clear if it represents a marker, a limited adaptive or pathological process [75].

The ECG abnormalities observed in *intracranial hemorrhage* may also influence clinical outcome. QTc prolongation correlated with insular cortex involvement, presence of intraventricular blood, and hydrocephalus on admission CT scans in patients with intracranial hemorrhage [81]. A case of a 58-year-old woman, with several episodes of self-terminating torsade de pointes (TdP) following nonspecific ST-T changes, and prolonged QT after brainstem hemorrhage, has been reported in the literature [82]. Maramattom et al. found premature ventricular contractions and QTc prolongation at 24 hours from admission, not related with the location, volume and side of the hemorrhage, nor with the presence of hydrocephalus, extraparenchymal extension or troponin T elevation [83].

It is uncertain whether ECG abnormalities are caused by the cerebrovascular event itself, considering that in the majority of studies patients' previous ECG data were unavailable [61]. Current management after stroke focuses mostly on the neurological function [62]. The QT interval and electrolyte levels should be monitored, and QT prolonging drugs should be avoided in patients with acute cerebrovascular events, especially for female patients with insular cortex lesions [61]. Multiple studies recommend continuous ECG monitoring, however, others believe that only severely QTc interval prolongation predicts cardiac complications [62]. Follow up studies with large sample sizes, considering previous arrhythmias and coronary heart disease, are needed, to establish the incidence of ventricular arrhythmias after stroke, and clear guidelines for clinicians approaching stroke patients with increased ventricular arrhythmia risk [62].

Goldberger et al. reported an unusual case of idiopathic acute *encephalopathy*, with persistent fever, refractory seizure, marked ventricular repolarization with bursts of torsade de pointes, diffuse ST elevations and Brugada-like pattern, treated with propofol [68].

Two mechanisms connecting cardiomyopathies and neurological diseases have been described: cardiomyopathies may either secondarily cause neurological disease or may represent the cardiac manifestation of a neurological disease, especially neuromuscular disorders [2]. Sudden cardiac death and ventricular arrhythmias occur mainly in neurological diseases causing hypertrophic cardiomyopathy (in adolescents and young adults), or dilated cardiomyopathy (among which syncope is a common clinical manifestation), or arrhythmogenic right ventricular dysplasia [2]. Takotsubo cardiomyopathy ("the broken heart" syndrome) was reported after stroke, subarachnoid bleeding, spontaneous intracerebral bleeding, *spinal injury and head trauma,* and the patients are prone to arrhythmias, heart failure or thrombus formation within the left ventricle during the acute phase [2]. *Inherited neuromuscular disorders* may predispose to premature ventricular contractions, monomorphic and polymorphic ventricular tachycardia and sudden cardiac death, due to degenerative changes in the myocardium [35]. Electrical abnormalities, including QTc and JTc dispersion (the difference between the longest and shortest JT interval duration), may be the earliest manifestation of cardiomyopathy in patients with *Emery-Dreifuss muscular dystrophy*, a hereditary muscle disorder characterized by slowly progressive muscle wasting and weakness, with humero-peroneal distribution [84]. QTc and JTc dispersions (QTcd, JTcd) reflect ventricular repolarization heterogeneities, due to diffuse fibrosis and fatty acid infiltration in Emery-Dreifuss muscular dystrophy, and if elevated, increase the risk of development of malignant ventricular arrhythmias via early afterdepolarization and reentry (polymorphic ventricular tachyarrhythmia), facilitated by intramural functional conduction blocks [84]. The mechanisms underlying sudden cardiac death in *myotonic dystrophy type 1* are: bradyarrhythmias due to cardiac conduction abnormalities, and the increased values of the QT variability index, demonstrating an important heart involvement, extended beyond the conduction system [85]. *Duchenne muscular dystrophy*, related to a mutation in the dystrophin gene, the most common neuromuscular disease, causes progressive proximal muscle weakness of the legs and pelvis and a loss of muscle mass. It affects also the heart (myocyte degeneration, fibrosis and fatty infiltration), impairing ventricular repolarization, causing autonomic dysfunction, QTc prolongation and increase of QT dispersion, as an independent risk factor for ventricular arrhythmias of Lown grade III or higher [86-88]. Late ventricular potentials were reported in patients with Duchenne muscular dystrophy (31%), indicating the presence of a substrate for reentry ventricular arrhythmias, associated with local myocardial fibrosis, and identifying patients at high risk for sudden cardiac death [89]. Cardiac involvement was also mentioned in other dystrophinopathies, due to the replacement of myocardium by connective tissue or fat, but it remains subclinical in Duchenne and *Becker muscular dystrophy* [86]. Patients with primary and secondary neuromuscular disorders need to be obligatorily screened for cardiac disease and ventricular arrhythmia risk, as soon as the neurological diagnosis is established, and cardiac investigations should be regularly repeated, especially in the case of severe cardiac involvement [2]. Once cardiac involvement occurs, the clinician should consider invasive electrophysiological studies and ICD implantation [35].

In *Parkinson's disease* factors affecting cardiac conduction may include intrinsic or iatrogenic autonomic disturbances, cardiovascular comorbidities (cardiac ischemia, ventricular hypertrophy), and electrolyte imbalances due to diuretics [90]. The most common prescribed drugs with QT prolonging effect were: Dromperidone, with antiemetic effect and also used to treat symptomatic postural hypotension, Citalopram, an antidepressant, and some antimicrobial agents (macrolides, azoles and fluoroquinolones) in a study conducted by Malek et al. [90]. Combining such drugs with some antipsychotics, tricyclic antidepressants, antihistamines and anti-retrovirals has additive influence on QT interval prolongation [90]. Large epidemiological studies emphasized the difficulties in detecting transient drug-induced ventricular arrhythmia in outpatient clinics, due to too few events, despite frequent syncope [91]. Oka et al considered that QTc intervals are closely related to autonomic nervous system dysfunction in patients with Parkinson's disease, related to the progression of the disease [92, 93]. Deguchi et al. found prolonged QTc intervals in patients with Parkinson's disease, reflecting the degeneration of cardioselective sympathetic and parasympathetic neurons [94]. Artifacts related to muscle tremor may affect ECGs in patients with Parkinson's disease, but methods were found to reduce noise and variance of QTc [95]. Drugs known to prolong the QT interval are often prescribed in patients with Parkinson's disease, and therapy should consider additional risk factors, especially comorbidities, autonomic dysfunction and degeneration of cardioselective neurons [90, 94].

Sudden unexpected death in *epilepsy* is probably caused by periictal cardiorespiratory alterations, such as central apnea, bradyarrhythmia, and neurogenic pulmonary edema, and ventricular arrhythmias [96, 97]. Sudden cardiac death in patients with seizure disorders is facilitated by associated cardiovascular diseases, pathologic cardiac repolarization, sympathovagal imbalance and therapy used to treat the disease [35, 96, 97]. A pathologic cardiac repolarization has been described in epileptic patients, with prolonged intercritical and periictal QT intervals, increased QT dispersion and shortened QTc after generalized tonic-clonic seizures, but fatal seizure-related ventricular arrhythmias are very rare [96]. On the other hand, no LVPs and significant standard ECG abnormalities were recorded in patients with newly diagnosed epilepsy, without clinical evidence of heart disease, three to nine months after therapy start, demonstrating lack of antiepileptic drugs induced electrocardiographic abnormalities [98]. Rejdak et al. reported abnormal SAECGs and late ventricular potentials in epilepsy patients, associated with disease duration, higher monthly seizure frequency, refractory epilepsy and tendency for higher number of generalized tonic-clonic seizures, polytherapy [99]. Data about intercritical QT intervals in epileptic patients are contradictory; it was found within normal limits, shorter or longer, and antiepileptic drugs and the ketogenic diet are potential confounders [96]. Transient dysfunction of cortical networks, as interictal epileptiform electroencephalographic discharges, can impair cardiac repolarization causing transient QTc prolongation [100]. Potential mechanisms of periictal QTc prolongation include cerebral dysregulation, ictal hypoxemia and hypercapnia, cardiorespiratory interactions, sympathetic stimulation, release of stress hormones and cardiac dysfunction [96, 101]. Generalized tonic-clonic seizures are a risk factor for sudden cardiac death, and cause QTc shortening due probably to seizure-related release of catecholamines, hyperkalemia, and acidosis [96]. The increased QT dispersion is explained by autonomic dysfunction with increased sympathetic tone, and subtle perivascular and interstitial fibrosis, which have been described in epilepsy [102, 103].

In order to reduce the risk of, or prevent, sudden cardiac death, 12-lead ECG should be performed in every patient with epilepsy, in order to identify those at high risk, and, therapy may include antiarrhythmic medication and implantation of cardiac combined pacemaker–defibrillator devices [96]. Cardiogenic syncope is often a difficult differential diagnosis for seizures, and long QT with recurrent syncope has been mistaken for epilepsy, and, epileptic seizures, probably due to cerebral hypoperfusion, have been described in patients with congenital long QT [96, 104]. Mutations of ionic channels could affect both heart and brain function, thereby leading to a susceptibility to epilepsy and cardiac arrhythmias [96].

8. Hematologic diseases and ventricular arrhythmia risk

Anemia and red blood cells transfusions have been associated with arrhythmias. Several electrocardiographic changes were previously mentioned in patients with *anemia*, including prolonged QT intervals, ST segment depression, inverted T waves, increased R amplitude after stress test [105]. Anemia was associated with prolonged QT intervals in hypertensive [106] and end stage renal disease patients [107], as well. Associations between the QT interval and serum ferritin level [108] and anisocytosis [106], respectively, were mentioned. Scheller et al. [109] reported a gradual prolongation of the QT and QTc interval in normovolemic anemia. Anemia may increase cardiac output and heart rate, may lead to eccentric left ventricular hypertrophy, activation of the sympathetic nervous system, stimulation of the renin angiotensin aldosterone system, and is closely associated with chronic inflammation and increased oxidative stress [106, 110]. Tissue hypoxia and changes in blood flow patterns due to low hemoglobin may play an atherogenic role [110]. The pathophysiological link between anemia and prolonged QT intervals and ventricular arrhythmia risk is, probably, hypoxia and decreased myocardial oxygen supply [106].

Jaja et al [111] reported a blunted autonomic cardiovascular response to changes in posture in patients with *sickle cell anemia*. Left ventricular systolic and diastolic dysfunction, increased

QTc intervals and QT dispersions and late ventricular potentials were found in patients with *beta-thalassemia*, a genetic cause of anemia, due to reduced synthesis of beta-globin chains [112, 113]. Several mechanisms explain increased sudden cardiac death in patients with thalassemia, including iron overload thalassemic cardiomyopathy, with patchy cardiac iron depostition (due to intensive blood transfusions), changes in calcium homeostasis, elevated prostaglandin E2 to prostacyclin ratio, increased interleukin 1 level and lipid peroxidation [106, 113, 114].

Athar et al. reported that packed red blood cells (PRBC) *transfusions* were independently associated with an increased risk of new onset cardiac arrhythmias and conduction abnormalities in patients with acute myocardial infarction [64]. Multiple factors contributed to the development of atrial fibrillation in the setting of acute myocardial infarction, including pericarditis, atrial ischemia, infarction, changes in autonomic tone, metabolic abnormalities, increased atrial pressures and inflammation [64]. The inflammatory process, exacerbated by PRBC transfusion, tissue hypoxia, exacerbations of cardiac ischemia and reinfarctions resulting from deficiencies in the ability of stored packed red blood cells to deliver oxygen to tissue, may explain the appearance of ventricular arrhythmias [64].

A significant correlation was found between QT dispersion and *platelet count* in healthy centenarians, hypothesizing that a reduced number of platelets and the maintenance of normal QT dispersion may contribute to the extreme longevity and protects centenarians from cardiovascular events [115].

Anthracyclines, used in therapy of patients with *hematological malignancies,* may have cardiotoxic effects, and the typical cardiac manifestations include cardiomyopathy, QT prolongation, ventricular ectopy and torsade de pointes [35, 116]. High intermittent doses and excessive cumulative doses increase the risk of cardiomyopathy and fatal arrhythmias, risk factors including age, female gender, hypertension, preexisting cardiac diseases, electrolyte imbalances, associated therapy with other QT prolonging drugs [35, 117]. Long term cardiac monitoring of patients is needed, in order to prevent sudden cardiac death and cardiac decompensation.

9. Conclusions

Sudden cardiac death, due to fatal ventricular arrhythmias, continues to be an important public health problem in developed countries. A high ventricular arrhythmia risk has been reported in several noncardiac diseases, including metabolic, liver, blood, neurological and psychiatric disorders. The most common mechanisms were: autonomic and electrolyte imbalances, ion channel remodeling, cardiomyopathies, increased oxidative stress and QT prolonging drugs. Most of the mentioned studies used standard 12-lead ECG and surrogate markers of ventricular arrhythmia risk (QT interval duration, QT dispersion and signal averaged ECG), but several papers reported ventricular arrhythmias, as well.

Considering that there are no guidelines for the prevention and therapy of arrhythmias appearing in most of extracardiac disorders, the present review highlighted important epidemiological and pathophysiological issues related to this topic.

Selected patients could benefit from electrocardiographic monitoring, specific therapy and avoidance of QT prolonging drugs, decreasing the burden of sudden cardiac death. Large follow up studies are needed, controlling for previous QT interval durations, arrhythmias, coronary heart disease and cardiovascular risk factors, in order to assess the prevalence of ventricular arrhythmias in noncardiac diseases, to identify further mechanisms and risk factors for arrhythmogenesis, and to elaborate clear guidelines for clinicians approaching the mentioned pathology.

Author details

Ioana Mozos*

Address all correspondence to: ioanamozos@umft.ro

"Victor Babes" University of Medicine and Pharmacy, Department of Functional Sciences, Timisoara, Romania

References

[1] Pollack ML. ECG Manifestations of Selected Extracardiac Diseases. Emerg MedClin. 2006;24:133-143.

[2] Finsterer J, Stöllberger C, Wahbi K. Cardiomyopathy in neurological disorders. Cardiovascular Pathology 2013; http://dx.doi.org/10.1016/j.carpath.2012.12.008

[3] Tereshchenko LG. Electrocardiogram as a screening tool in the general population: A strategic review. J Electrocardiol. 2013;doi:10.1016/j.jelectrocard.2013.07.005

[4] Rautaharju PM, Surawicz B, Gettes LS, et al. AHA/ACC/HRS recommendations for the standardization and interpretation of the electrocardiogram. Part IV: The ST segment, T and U waves, and the QT interval: A scientific statement from the American Heart association Electrocardiography and Arrhythmias Committee, Council on Clinical Cardiology; the American College of Cardiology Foundation; and the Heart Rhythm Society; Endorsed by the International Society for Computerized Electrocardiology. Circulation 2009;119:e241-e250.

[5] Mozoş I, Şerban C and Mihăescu R. Late Ventricular Potentials in Cardiac and Extracardiac Diseases. In: Breijo- Marquez FR (ed). Cardiac Arrhythmias - New Considerations. Rjeka:InTech; 2012, p227-256. Available from: http://www.intechopen.com/books/cardiac-arrhythmias-new-considerations/late-ventricular-potentials-in-cardiac-and-extracardiac-diseases (accessed 15 September, 2013).

[6] Su L, Borov S, Zrenner B. 12-lead Holter electrocardiography. Review of the literature and clinical application update. Herzschrittmacherther Elektophysiol. 2013;24(2): 92-6.

[7] Priori SG, Aliot E, Blomstrom-Lundqvist C, et al. Task Force on Sudden Cardiac Death of the European Society of Cardiology. Task Force Report. Eur Heart J. 2001;22(16):1374-1450.

[8] Liu YB, Wu CC, Lu LS, et al. Sympathetic Nerve Sprouting, electrical remodeling, and increased vulnerability to ventricular fibrillation in hypercholesterolemic rabbits. Circ Res. 2003;92:1145-1152.

[9] Kumar P, Goyal M, Agarwal JL. Effect of L-arginine on electrocardiographic changes induced by hypercholesterolemia and isoproterenol in rabbits. Indian Pacing Electrophysiol. 2009;9(1):45-52.

[10] Liu YB, Lee YT, Pak HN, et al. Effects of simvastatin on cardiac neural and electrophysiologic remodeling in rabbits with hypercholesterolemia. Heart Rhythm 2009; 61(1):69-75.

[11] Burke AP, Farb A, Malcom GT, et al. Coronary risk factors and plaque morphology in men with coronary disease who died suddenly. N Engl J Med. 1997;336(18): 1276-82.

[12] Kostapanos MS, Liberopoulos EN, Goudevenos JA, et al. Do statins have an antiarrhythmic activity? Cardiovasc Res. 2007;75(1):10-20.

[13] Gualdiero P, Esposito K, Ciotola M, et al. (2002). Simvastatin normalizes QTc dispersion and reduces ventricular electrical instability in isolated hypercholesterolemia. J Endocrinol Invest. 2002;25:RC16-RC18.

[14] Szabo Z, Harangi M, Lörincz I, et al. Effect of hyperlipidemia on QT dispersion in patients without ischemic heart disease. Can J Cardiol. 2005;21(10):847-850.

[15] Paragh G, Nagy JT, Szondy E, et al. Immunomodulating effect of low density lipoprotein on human monocytes. Clin Exp Immunol. 1986;64:665-672.

[16] Mozos I & Hancu M. High serum cholesterol and electrical instability in patients with an old myocardial infarction. Atherosclerosis Supplements 2010;11(2):109-222.

[17] Chu CS, Lee KT, Lee ST, et al. Effects of atorvastatin on ventricular late potentials and ventricular late potentials and repolarization dispersion in patients with hypercholesterolemia. Kaohsiung J Med Sci. 2007;23:217–24.

[18] Abuissa H, O'Keefe JH, Bybee KA.Statins as anti-arrhythmics: a systematic review part II: effects on risk of ventricular arrhythmias. Clin Cardiol. 2009;23(10):542-52.

[19] Duflou J, Virmani R, Rabin L, et al. Sudden death as a result of heart disease in morbid obesity. Am Heart J. 1995;130:306-13.

[20] Lalani AP, Kanna B, John J, et al. Abnormal Signal-Averaged Electrocardiogram (SAECG) in Obesity. Obesity Research 2000;8(1):20-28.

[21] Mizia-Stec K, Mandecki T, Zahorska-Markiewicz B, et al. The QT interval dispersion and ventricular late potential in obese women. Pol Merkur Lekarski. 2000;8(44):84-6.

[22] Gamal A, Gallagher D, Nawras A, et al. Effects of obesity on QT, RR, and QTc intervals. Am J Cardiol. 1995;75:956-959.

[23] Carella MJ, Mantz SL, Rovner DR, et al.Obesity, adiposity, and lengthening of the QT interval: improvement after weight loss. Int J Obes Realat Metab Disord. 1996;20:938-942.

[24] Queen SR, Smulevitz B, Rentfro AR, et al. Electrocardiographic abnormalities among Mexican Americans: correlations with diabetes, obesity, and the metabolic syndrome. World J Cardiovasc Dis. 2012;2(2):50-56.

[25] Alexander JK. The cardiomyopathy of obesity. Prog Cardiovasc Dis.1985;28:325-34.

[26] Bharati S & Lev M. Cardiac conduction system involvement in sudden death of obese young people. Am Heart J. 1995;129:273-81.

[27] Schunkert H. Obesity and target organ damage: the heart. International Journal of Obesity 2002;26 (Suppl 4):S15 – S20.

[28] Mozos I, Hancu M, Chiulan C, et al. Aspects of Electrical Instability in Obese Chronic Myocardial Infarction Patients, In: Strbak V (ed). Joint Meeting of the Slovak Physiological Society, the Physiological Society and the Federation of European Physiological Societies. Bratislava (Slovak Republic), September 11-14, 2007. Bologna, Italy: Medimond International Proceedings. Monduzzi Editore; 2007. p.95-98.

[29] Pontiroli AE, Merlotti C, Veronelli A, et al. Effect of weight loss on sympatho-vagal balance in subjects with grade-3 obesity: restrictive surgery versus hypocaloric diet. Acta Diabetol. 2013;doi: 10.1007/s00592-013-0454-1

[30] Takimoto Y, Yoshiuchi K, Kumano H, et al. Bulimia nervosa and abnormal cardiac repolarization. J Psychosom Res. 2006;60(1):105-7.

[31] Buchanan R, Ngwira J, Amsha K. Prolonged QT interval in bulimia nervosa. BMJ Case Reports 2011;doi: 10.1136/bcr.01.2011.3780.

[32] Krantz MJ, Sabel AL, Sagar U, et al. Factors influencing QT prolongation in patients hospitalized with severe anorexia nervosa. Gen Hosp Psychiatry. 2012;34(2):173-7.

[33] Pacher P, Ungvari Z, Nanasi PP, et al. Electrophysiological changes in rat ventricular and atrial myocardium at different stages of experimental diabetes. Acta Physiol Scand. 1999;166(1):7-13.

[34] Kowalewski MA, Urban M, Florys B, et al. Late potentials: Are they related to cardiovascular complications in children with type 1 diabetes? J Diabetes Complications. 2002;16(4):263-270.

[35] Zipes D, Camm AJ, Borggrefe M et al. ACC/AHA/ESC 2006 guidelines for management of patients with ventricular arrhythmias and the prevention of sudden cardiac death: a report of the American College of Cardiology/American Heart Association Task Force and the European Society of Cardiology Committee for Practice Guidelines. Europace 2006;8:746-836.

[36] Lu Z, Jiang YP, Wu CY, et al. Increased persistent sodium current due to decreased PI3K signaling contributes to QT prolongation in the diabetic heart. Diabetes 2013;doi: 10.2337/db13-0420

[37] Kumar R, Fisher M, Macfarlane PW. Diabetes and the QT interval: time for debate. Br J Diabetes Vasc Dis. 2004;4:146-50.

[38] Veglio M, Borra M, Stevens LK, et al. The relationship between QTc interval prolongation and diabetic complications: the EURODIABIDDM Complication Study Group. Diabetologia 1999;42:68-75.

[39] Marfella R, Nappo F, De Angelis L, et al.The effect of acute hyperglycemia on QTc duration in healthy men. Diabetologia 2000;43:571-5.

[40] Li X, Ren H, Xu ZR, et al. Prevalence and risk factors of prolonged QTc interval among Chinese patients with type 2 diabetes. Exp Diabetes Res. 2012;doi: 10.1155/2012/234084

[41] Marfella R, Siniscalchi M, Esposito K, et al. Effects of stress hyperglycemia on acute myocardial infarction: role of inflammatory immune process in functional cardiac outcome. Diabetes Care 2003;26(11):3129-35.

[42] Sanjuan R, Nunez J, Blasco ML, et al.Prognostic implications of stress hyperglycemia in acute ST elevation myocardial infarction. Prospective observational study. Rev Esp Cardiol. 2011;64(3):201-7.

[43] Laitinen T, Lyyra-Laitinen T, Huopio H, et al. Electrocardiographic alterations during hyperinsulinemic hypoglycemia in healthy subjects. Ann Noninvasive Electrocardiol. 2008; 13:97-105.

[44] Beom JW, Kim JM, Chung EJ, et al. Corrected QT interval prolongation during severe hypoglycemia without hypokalemia in patients with type 2 diabetes. Diabetes Metab J. 2013;37:190-195.

[45] Tattersall RB, Gill GV. Unexplained deaths of type 1 diabetic patients. Diabet Med. 1991;8:49-58.

[46] Wong F. Cirrhotic cardiomyopathy. Hepatol Int. 2009;3:294-304.

[47] Genovesi S, Prata Pizzala M, Pozzi M, et al. QT interval prolongation and decreased heart rate variability in cirrhotic patients: relevance of hepatic venous pressure gradient and serum calcium. Clin Sci. 2009;116:851-9.

[48] Mozos I, Costea C, Serban C, et al. Factors associated with a prolonged QT interval in liver cirrhosis patients. J Electrocardiol. 2011;44:105-108.

[49] Bernardi M, Maggioli C, Dibra V, et al. QT interval prolongation in liver cirrhosis: innocent bystander or serious threat? Expert Rev Gastroenterol Hepatol. 2012;6(1): 57-66.

[50] Day CP, James OF, Butler TJ, et al. QT prolongation and sudden cardiac death in patients with alcoholic liver disease. Lancet 1993;341:1423-1428.

[51] Kempler P, Szalay F, Varadi A, et al. Prolongation of the QTc-interval reflects the severity of autonomic neuropathy in primary biliary cirrhosis and in other non-alcoholic liver diseases. Z Gastroenterol. 1993;31(Suppl 2):96-8.

[52] Zamirian M, Tavassoli M, Aghasadeghi K. Corrected QT interval and QT dispersion in cirrhotic patients before and after liver transplantation. Arch Iran Med. 2012;15(6): 375-377.

[53] Ytting H, Henriksen JH, Fuglsang S, et al. Prolonged Q-Tc interval in mild portal hypertensive cirrhosis. J Hepatol. 2005;43(4):637-44.

[54] Moller S, Hove JD, Dixen U, et al. New insights into cirrhotic cardiomyopathy. Int J Cardiol. 2013;167(4):1101-1108.

[55] Bal JS, Thuluvath PJ.Prolongation of QTc interval: relationship with etiology and severity of liver disease, mortality and liver transplantation. Liver Int. 2003;23(4):243-8.

[56] Trevisani F, Di Micoli A, Zambruni A, et al. QT interval prolongation by acute gastrointestinal bleeding in patients with cirrhosis. Liver Int. 2012;32(10):1510-5.

[57] Zambruni A, Trevisani F, Caraceni P, et al. Cardiac electrophysiological abnormalities in patients with cirrhosis. J Hepatol. 2006;44:994-1002.

[58] Baik SK, Fouad TR, Lee SS. Cirrhotic cardiomyopathy. Orphanet J Rare Dis. 2007; 2 : 2-15.

[59] Almawardy R, Elhammady W, Mousa N, et al. Is combination therapy for chronic hepatitis C toxic for cardiac function? Hepat Mon. 2012;12(8):6254.

[60] Basile AM, Di Carlo A, Lamassa M, et al. Selective risk factors profiles and outcomes among patients with stroke and history of prior myocardial infarction. The European Community Stroke Project. J Neurol Sci. 2008;264:87-92.

[61] Katsanos AH, Korantzopoulos P, Tsivgoulis G, et al. Electrocardiographic abnormalities and cardiac arrhythmias in structural brain lesions. Int J Cardiol. 2013;167: 328-334.

[62] Koppikar S, Baranchuk A, Guzman JC, et al. Stroke and ventricular arrhythmias. Int J Cardiol. 2013; http://dx.doi.org/10.1016/j.ijcard.2013.03.058

[63] Dennis MS, Burn JP, Sandercock PA, et al. Long-term survival after first-ever stroke: the Oxfordshire Community Stroke Project. Stroke 1993;24:796-800.

[64] Athar MK, Bagga M, Nair N, et al. Risk of cardiac arrhythmias and conduction abnormalities in patients with acute myocardial infarction receiving packed red blood cell transfusions. J Clin Care. 2011;26:335-341.

[65] Dogan A, Tunc E, Ozturk M, et al. Electrocardiographic changes in patients with ischemic stroke and their prognostic importance. J Clin Pract. 2004;58(5):436-440.

[66] Mozos I, Costea C, Costea S. Intervalul QT la pacienţii cu accident vascular cerebral. Infomedica 2008;1(143):32-36.

[67] Sommargren CE. Electrocardiographic abnormalities in patients with subarachnoid hemorrhage. Am J Crit Care. 2002;11(1):48–56.

[68] Goldberger ZD, Creutzfeldt CJ, Goldberger AL. Catastrophic neurologic syndrome with dramatic ECG changes. J Electrocardiol. 2013;doi: 10.1016/j.ielectrocard. 2013.07.014

[69] Kallmunzer B, Breuer L, Kahl N, et al. Serious cardiac arrhythmias after stroke: incidence, time course, and predictors—a systematic, prospective analysis. Stroke 2012;43: 2892–7.

[70] Sander D, Winbeck K, Klingelhofer J, et al. Prognostic relevance of pathological sympathetic activation after acute thromboembolic stroke. Neurology 2001;57(5):833–8.

[71] Oppenheimer SM, Kedem G,MartinWM. Left-insular cortex lesions perturb cardiac autonomic tone in humans. Clin Auton Res. 1996;6:131–40.

[72] Wong KYK, Mac Walter RS, Douglas D, et al. Long QTc predicts future cardiac death in stroke survivors. Heart 2003;89:377–381.

[73] Stead LG, Gilmore RM, Bellolio MF, et al. Prolonged QTc as a predictor of mortality in acute ischemic stroke. J Stroke Cerebrovasc Dis. 2009;18(6):469–74.

[74] Frangiskakis JM, Hravnak M, Crago EA, et al. Ventricular arrhythmia risk after subarachnoid hemorrhage. Neurocrit Care. 2009;10(3):287–94.

[75] Soliman EZ, Howard G, Cushman M, et al. Prolongation of QTc and Risk of Stroke. The REGARDS (REasons for Geographic and Racial Differences in Stroke) Study. JACC. 2012;59(16):1460-67.

[76] Di Pasquale G, Pinelli G, Andreoli A, et al. Holter detection of cardiac arrhythmias in intracranial subarachnoid hemorrhage. Am J Cardiol. 1987;59:596–600.

[77] Festa A, D'Agostino R, Rautaharju P, et al. Is QT interval a marker of subclinical atherosclerosis in nondiabetic subjects? The Insulin Resistance Atherosclerosis Study (IRAS). Stroke 1999;30:1566 –71.

[78] Strohmer B,Pichler M, Iqlseder B, et al. Relationship of QT interval duration with carotid intima media thickness in a clinically healthy population undergoing cardiovascular risk screening. J Intern Med. 2005;257(3):238-46.

[79] Maebuchi D, Arima H, Ninomiya T et al. Arterial stiffness and QT interval prolongation in a general population: The Hisayama study. Hypertension Res. 2008;31:1339-45.

[80] Mozos I, Filimon L. The QT interval, arterial stiffness, endothelial function and vascular age. J Electrocardiol. 2013;46:e20.

[81] Van Bree MD, Roos YB, van der Bilt IA, et al. Prevalence and characterization of ECG abnormalities after intracerebral hemorrhage. Neurocrit Care 2010;1:50–5.

[82] Chao CL, Chen WJ, Wu CC, et al.Torsade de pointes and T-wave alternans in a patient with brainstem hemorrhage. Int J Cardiol. 1995;51(2):199–201.

[83] Maramattom BV, Manno EM, Fulgham JR, et al. Clinical importance of cardiac troponin release and cardiac abnormalities in patients with supratentorial cerebral hemorrhages. Mayo Clin Proc. 2006;81(2):192–6.

[84] Russo V, Rago A, Politano L, et al. Increased dispersion of ventricular repolarization in Emery Dreifuss muscular dystrophy patients. Med Sci Monit. 2012;18(11):CR643-647

[85] Magri D, Piccirillo G, Bucci E, et al. Increased temporal dispersion of myocardial repolarization in myotonic dystrophy type 1: beyond the cardiac conduction system. Int J Cardiol. 2012;156(3):259-64.

[86] Finsterer J, Stöllberger C. The heart in human dystrophinopathies. Cardiology 2003;99(1):1-19.

[87] Yotsukura M, Yamamoto A, Kajiwara T, et al. QT dispersion in patients with Duchenne-type progressive muscular dystrophy. Am Heart J. 1999;137:672-7.

[88] Santos MAB, de Assis Costa F, Ferreira Travessa A, et al. Distrofia Muscular de Duchenne: analisis electrocardiografica de 131 pacientes. Arq Bras Cardiol. 2010;94(4):602-606.

[89] Kubo M, Matsuoka S, Taguchi Y, et al. Clinical significance of late potentials in patients with Duchenne muscular dystrophy. Pediatr Cardiol. 1993;14(4):214-9.

[90] Malek NM, Grosset KA, Stewart D, et al. Prescription of drugs with potential adverse effects on cardiac conduction in Parkinson's disease. Parkinsonism Relat Disord. 2013; 19(6):586-9.

[91] Woodford H, Walker R. Emergency hospital admissions in idiopathic Parkinson's disease. Mov Disord. 2005;20:104e8.

[92] Oka H, Mochio S, Sato H, et al. Prolongation of QTc interval in patients with Parkinson's disease. Eur Neurol. 1997;37(3):186-9.

[93] Oka H, Mochio S, Inoue K. Relation between autonomic dysfunction and progression of Parkinson's disease. Rinsho Shinkeigaku 2001:41(6):283-8.

[94] Deguchi K, Sasaki I, Tsukaguchi M, et al. Abnormalities of rate-corrected QT intervals in Parkinson's disease e a comparison with multiple system atrophy and progressive supranuclear palsy. J Neurol Sci. 2002;199(1e2):31e7.

[95] Bloomfield DM. Evaluating QTc in patients with advanced Parkinson's disease: Overcoming artefacts. Clin Pharmacol Ther. 2009;85(4):365-6.

[96] Surges R, Taggart P, Sander JW, et al. Too long or too short? New insights into abnormal cardiac repolarization in people with chronic epilepsy and its potential role in sudden unexpected death. Epilepsia 2010;51(5):738-744.

[97] Lotufo PA, Valiengo L, Bensenor IM, et al. A systematic review and meta-analysis of heart rate variability in epilepsy and antiepileptic drugs. Epilepsia 2012;53(2):272-82.

[98] Svalheim S, Aurlien D, Amlie JP, et al. Signal-averaged and standard electrocardiography in patients with newly diagnosed epilepsy. Epilepsy Behav. 2012;25(4):543-5.

[99] Rejdak K, Rubaj A, Glowniak A, et al. (2011). Analysis of ventricular late potentials in signal-averaged ECG of people with epilepsy. Epilepsia 2011;52(11):2118-24.

[100] Tavernor SJ, Brown SW, Tavernor RM, et al.Electrocardiograph QT lengthening associated with epileptiform EEG discharges–a role in sudden unexplained death in epilepsy? Seizure 1996;5:79–83.

[101] Damasceno DD, Ferreira AJ, Doretto MC, et al. Cardiovascular dysautonomia after seizures induced by maximal electroshock in Wistar rats. Seizure 2012;21(9):711-6.

[102] Schraeder PL, Lathers CM. Cardiac neural discharge and epileptogenic activity in the cat: an animal model for unexplained death. Life Sci. 1983;32:1371–1382.

[103] Natelson BH, Suarez RV, Terrence CF, et al. Patients with epilepsy who die suddenly have cardiac disease. Arch Neurol. 1998;55:857–860.

[104] Betge S, Schulze-Bahr E, Fitzek C, et al. Long-QT-Syndrom als Differenzialdiagnose einer Grand-Mal-Epilepsie. Fallbericht, Stammbaum, Therapieoptionen und Literaturübersicht. Nervenarzt 2006;77:1210–1217.

[105] Stanojevic M, Stankov S. Electrocardiographic changes in patients with chronic anemia. Srp Arh Celok Lek. 1998;126(11-12):461-6.

[106] Mozos I, Serban C, Mihaescu R. Anemia and the QT interval in hypertensive patients International Journal of Collaborative Research on Internal Medicine and Public Health 2012;4(12):2084-2091.

[107] Ijoma CK, Ulasi II, Anisiuba BC. Anemia predicts prolonged QT interval in predialysis chronic kidney disease patients. The Internet Journal of Cardiovascular Research 2010:7(1): doi: 10.5580/1d12.

[108] Khode VH, Kammar KF. QTc changes in non-pregnant females with severe iron deficiency anaemia. Journal of Clinical and Diagnostic Research 2012;6(5):777-779.

[109] Scheller B, Pipa G, Kertscho H, et al. Low hemoglobin levels during normovolemia are associated with electrocardiographic changes in pigs. Shock 2011;34(4):375-81.

[110] Zoppini G, Targher G, Chonchol M, et al. Anemia, in dependent of chronic kidney disease, predicts all-cause and cardiovascular mortality in type 2 diabetic patients. Atherosclerosis 2010;10:575-580.

[111] Jaja ST, Kehinde MO, Ogungbemi SI. Cardiac and autonomic responses to change in posture or vitamin C supplementation in sickle cell anemia subjects. Pathophysiology 2008;15:25-30.

[112] Garadah TS, Kassab S, Mahdi N, et al. QTc interval and QT dispersion in patients with thalassemia major: electrocardiographic (EKG) and echocardiographic evaluation. Clinical Medicine Insights: Cardiology 2010;4:31-37.

[113] Isma' eel H, Shamseddeen W, Taher A, et al. Ventricular late potentials among thalassemia patients. Int J Cardiol. 2007;132(3):453-5.

[114] Lekawanvijit S & Chattipakorn N. Iron overload thalassemic cardiomyopathy: Iron status assessment and mechanisms of mechanical and electrical disturbance due to iron toxicity. Can J Cardiol. 2009;25(4):213-218.

[115] Gangemi S, Basile G, Merendino RA, et al. Lower platelet count in healthy centenarians correlates with dispersion on the QT interval. Aging Clin Exp Res. 2004;16(2): 169-71.

[116] Mornos C, Petrescu L. Early detection of anthracycline-mediated cardiotoxicity: the value of considering both global longitudinal left ventricular strain and twist. Can J Pharmacol. 2013;91(8):601-7.

[117] Arbel Y, Swartzon M, Justo D. QT prolongation and Torsades de Pointes in patients previously treated with Anthracyclines. Anti-Cancer Drugs 2007;18:493-498.

Chapter 5

Treatment of Ventricular Arrhythmias

Wilbert S. Aronow

Additional information is available at the end of the chapter

http://dx.doi.org/10.5772/57545

1. Introduction

The presence of 3 or more consecutive ventricular premature complexes (VPCs) on an electrocardiogram is ventricular tachycardia (VT) [1, 2]. VT is sustained if it lasts ≥30 seconds and nonsustained if its lasts <30 seconds [2]. Complex ventricular arrhythmias (VA) are VT or paired, multiform, or frequent VPCs. This author diagnoses frequent VPCs if there are an average of ≥30/hour on a 24-hour ambulatory electrocardiogram (AECG) or ≥6/minute on a 1-minute rhythm strip of an electrocardiogram (ECG) [2, 3]. Simple VA are infrequent VPCs and no complex forms.

The prevalence of nonsustained VT diagnosed by 24-hour AECGs varied from 2% to 13% in older persons without cardiovascular disease [1, 4-7], was 9% in 385 older men and 8% in 806 older women with hypertension, valvular disease, or cardiomyopathy [7], and was 16% in 395 older men and 15% in 771 older women with coronary artery disease (CAD) [7]. The prevalence of complex VA in older persons in these studies varied from 16% to 50% in older persons without cardiovascular disease [1, 4-7], was 54% in older men and 55% in older women with hypertension, valvular disease, or cardiomyopathy [7], and was 69% in older men and 68% in older women with CAD [7].

In 104 older persons without cardiovascular disease, complex VA were present on 24-hour AECGs in 33% of persons and on 1-minute rhythm strips in 2% of persons [3]. In 843 older persons, with cardiovascular disease, complex VA were present on 24-hour AECGs in 55% of persons and on 1-minute rhythm strips in 4% of persons [3].

In persons with cardiovascular disease, those with an abnormal left ventricular (LV) ejection fraction [8], with echocardiographic LV hypertrophy [9], or with silent myocardial ischemia [10] have a higher prevalence of VT and of complex VA than those with normal LV ejection fraction, normal LV mass, and no myocardial ischemia.

INTECH
open science | open minds

© 2014 Aronow; licensee InTech. This is a paper distributed under the terms of the Creative Commons Attribution License (http://creativecommons.org/licenses/by/3.0), which permits unrestricted use, distribution, and reproduction in any medium, provided the original work is properly cited.

2. Prognosis of ventricular arrhythmias

In the Baltimore Longitudinal Study of Aging, nonsustained VT or complex VA were not associated with new
coronary events at 10-year follow-up of 98 persons without heart disease [11]. In this study, exercise-induced nonsustained VT was not associated with new coronary events at 2-year follow-up in persons without heart disease [12]. At 5.6-year follow-up in this study, exercise-induced frequent or repetitive VPCs also were not associated with new coronary events in persons without heart disease [13].

Nonsustained VT or complex VA diagnosed by 24-hour AECGs were not associated with new coronary events at 2-year follow-up in 76 persons without heart disease [14] and were not associated with primary ventricular fibrillation (VF) or sudden cardiac death in 86 persons without heart disease [15]. Complex VA diagnosed by 24-hour AECGs or by 12-lead ECGs with 1-minute rhythm strips were also not associated with new coronary events at 39-month follow-up in 104 persons without heart disease [3]. Nonsustained VT or complex VA diagnosed by 24-hour AECGs were not associated with new coronary events at 45-month follow-up of 135 men and at 47-month follow-up of 297 women without cardiovascular disease [7].

Because nonsustained VT or complex VA are not associated with new coronary events in persons without heart disease, asymptomatic nonsustained VT or complex VA in persons without heart disease should not be treated with antiarrhythmic drugs. Because simple VA in persons with heart disease are not associated with new coronary events [3, 7, 11, 14, 15], simple VA in older persons with heart disease should not be treated with antiarrhythmic drugs.

However, patients with VT (sustained or nonsustained) or with complex VA associated with heart disease are at increased risk for developing new coronary events, primary VF, and sudden cardiac death [3, 7, 11, 14-19].

3. Medical therapy

Underlying causes of complex VA should be treated, if possible. Therapy of congestive heart failure (CHF), digitalis toxicity, hypokalemia, hypomagnesemia, hypertension, LV dysfunction, LV hypertrophy, myocardial ischemia by anti-ischemic drugs such as beta blockers or by coronary revascularization, hypoxia, and other conditions may abolish or decrease complex VA. Persons should not smoke or drink alcohol and should avoid drugs that may cause or increase complex VA.

CAD should be treated with aspirin [20-23], with beta blockers [23-28], with angiotensin-converting enzyme (ACE) inhibitors [23, 28-33], and with 3-hydroxy-3-methylglutaryl coenzyme A reductase inhibitors (statins) [23, 34-40] unless there are contraindications to these drugs. The serum low-density lipoprotein (LDL) cholesterol level should be reduced ≥ 50% by high-dose statins (atorvastatin 40to 80 mg daily or rosuvastatin 20 to 40 mg daily) [40].

Age-related physiologic changes may affect absorption, distribution, metabolism, and excretion of cardiovascular drugs [41]. Numerous physiologic changes with aging affect pharmacodynamics with alterations in end-organ responsiveness to cardiovascular drugs [41]. Drug interactions between antiarrhythmic drugs and other cardiovascular drugs are common [41]. There are also important drug-disease interactions [41]. Class I antiarrhythmic drugs have an unacceptable proarrhythmia rate in patients with heart disease and should be avoided. Class III antiarrhythmic drugs should also be used with caution in patients with heart disease since multiple factors may increase proarrhythmia. Except for beta blockers, all antiarrhythmic drugs may cause torsades de pointes (VT with polymorphous appearance associated with prolonged QT interval).

Class I antiarrhythmic drugs are sodium channel blockers. Class Ia antiarrhythmic drugs have intermediate channel kinetics and prolong repolarization. These drugs include quinidine, procainamide, and disopyramide. Class Ib antiarrhythmic drugs have rapid channel kinetics and slightly shorten repolarization. These drugs include lidocaine, mexilitine, tocainide, and phenytoin. Class Ic drugs have slow channel kinetics and have little effect on repolarization. These drugs include encainide, flecainide, moricizine, propafenone, and lorcainide. None of the Class I antiarrhythmic drugs have been found in controlled, clinical trials to reduce sudden cardiac death, total cardiac death, or total mortality.

The International Mexilitine and Placebo Antiarrhythmic Coronary Trial (IMPACT) was a prospective, double-blind, randomized study in survivors of myocardial infarction (MI) in whom 317 persons were randomized to mexilitine and 313 persons to placebo [42]. At 1-year follow-up, mortality was 7.6% for mexilitine-treated patients versus 4.8% for placebo-treated patients [42].

The Cardiac Arrhythmia Suppression Trial (CAST) I was a prospective, double-blind, randomized study in survivors of MI with asymptomatic or mildly symptomatic VA in which 730 patients were randomized to encainide or flecainide and 725 patients to placebo [43]. Adequate suppression of VA by encainide or flecainide was needed before randomization. Despite adequate suppression of VA, at 10-month follow-up, encainide and flecainide significantly increased mortality from arrhythmia or cardiac arrest 3.6 times and significantly increased total mortality 2.5 times[43). Older age increased the likelihood of adverse events, including death, in patients treated with encainide and flecainide[44].

CAST II was a prospective, double-blind, randomized study in survivors of MI with asymptomatic or mildly symptomatic VA in which 581 patients were randomized to moricizine and 574 patients to placebo. [45]. Adequate suppression of VA by moricizine was required before randomization. At 18-month follow-up, the mortality from arrhythmia or cardiac arrest was 8.4% for patients treated with moricizine and 7.3% for patients treated with placebo [45]. The 2-year survival rate was 81.7% for patients treated with moricizine and 85.6% for patients treated with placebo [45]. Older age increased the likelihood of adverse events, including death, in patients receiving moricizine [44].

Aronow et al [46] performed a prospective study in 406 persons with heart disease (58% with prior MI) and asymptomatic complex VA diagnosed by 24-hour AECGs. The prevalence of nonsustained VT was 20%. The prevalence of an abnormal ejection fraction was 32%. The incidence of adverse effects causing cessation of drug was 48% for quinidine and 55% for procainamide. At 24-month follow-up, the incidences of sudden cardiac death, total cardiac death, and of total death were not significantly different in persons treated with quinidine or procainamide or with no antiarrhythmic drug [46]. The incidence of total mortality was 65% for persons treated with quinidine or procainamide and 63% for persons treated with no antiarrhythmic drug. Quinidine or procainamide did not decrease sudden cardiac death, total cardiac death, or total death in comparison with no antiarrhythmic drug in older patients with ischemic or nonischemic heart disease, abnormal or normal LV ejection fraction, and presence versus absence of VT [46].

Moosvi et al [47] performed a retrospective analysis of the effect of empiric antiarrhythmic therapy in 209 resuscitated out-of-hospital cardiac arrest patients with CAD. Of the 209 patients, 48 received quinidine, 45 received procainamide, and 116 received no antiarrhythmic drug. The 2-year sudden death survival was 69% for quinidine-treated patients, 69% for procainamide-treated patients, and 89% for patients treated with no antiarrhythmic drug [47]. The 2-year total survival was 61% for quinidine-treated patients, 57% for procainamide-treated patients, and 71% for patients treated with no antiarrhythmic drug [47].

Hallstrom et al [48] performed a retrospective analysis of the effect of antiarrhythmic drug use in 941 patients resuscitated from prehospital cardiac arrest attributable to VF between 1970 and 1985. Quinidine was given to 19% of patients, procainamide to 18% of patients, beta blockers to 28% of patients, and no antiarrhythmic drug to 39% of patients. There was a 17% increased incidence of death or recurrent cardiac arrest in patients treated with quinidine or procainamide versus no antiarrhythmic drug. Survival was 57% worse for patients treated with procainamide than for patients treated with quinidine [48].

A meta-analysis of 6 double-blind studies of 808 patients with chronic atrial fibrillation who underwent direct-current cardioversion to sinus rhythm showed that the mortality at one year was higher in patients treated with quinidine (2.9%) than in patients treated with placebo (0.8%) [49]. Of 1, 330 patients in the Stroke Prevention in Atrial Fibrillation Study, 127 were receiving quinidine, 57 procainamide, 15 disopyramide, 34 flecainide, 20 encainide, and 7 amiodarone [50]. The adjusted relative risk of cardiac mortality was 1.8 times higher and the adjusted relative risk of arrhythmic death was 2.1 times higher in patients receiving antiarrhythmic drugs [50]. In patients with a history of CHF, the adjusted relative risk of cardiac death was 3.3 times higher and the adjusted relative risk of arrhythmic death was 5.8 times higher in patients receiving antiarrhythmic drugs[50].

Morganroth and Goin [51] performed a meta-analysis of 4 randomized, double-blind controlled trials lasting 2 to 12 weeks in which quinidine (n=502) was compared with flecainide (n=141), mexiletine (n=246), tocainide (n=67), and propafenone (n=53) in the treatment of complex VA. There was an increased risk of mortality in patients treated with quinidine compared with patients treated with the other antiarrhythmic drugs (absolute risk increase = 1.6%) [51].

Teo et al [52] analyzed 59 randomized controlled trials of 23, 229 patients that investigated use of Class I antiarrhythmic drugs after MI. The Class I drugs investigated included quinidine, procainamide, disopyramide, imipramine, moricizine, lidocaine, tocainide, phenytoin, mexiletine, aprindine, encainide, and flecainide. Mortality was 14% higher in patients receiving Class I antiarrhythmic drugs than in patients receiving no antiarrhythmic drugs. None of the 59 studies demonstrated that use of a Class I antiarrhythmic drug decreased mortality in postinfarction patients [52].On the basis of these data, no Class I antiarrhythmic drugs should be used for the treatment of VT or complex VA.

Calcium channel blockers are not useful in treatment of complex VA. Although verapamil can terminate a left septal fascicular VT, hemodynamic collapse can occur if intravenous verapamil is given to patients with the more common forms of reentry VT. Teo et al [52] analyzed randomized controlled trials of 20, 342 patients that investigated the use of calcium channel blockers after MI. Mortality was insignificantly 4% higher in patients receiving calcium channel blockers than in patients receiving no antiarrhythmic drugs [52]. On the basis of these data, no calcium channel blockers should be used in the treatment of VT or complex VA.

Teo et al [52] analyzed 55 randomized controlled trials comprising 53, 268 patients that investigated use of beta blockers after MI. Mortality was significantly reduced 19% in patients receiving beta blockers [52]. The decrease in mortality after MI in persons treated with beta blockers was due to both a reduction in sudden cardiac death and recurrent MI [24-27, 53].

The Beta Blocker Heart Attack Trial was a double-blind, randomized study of 3, 290 patients after MI [53-55]. At 25-month follow-up, propranolol decreased sudden cardiac death by 28% in patients with complex VA and by 16% in patients without complex VA. Propranolol significantly reduced total mortality by 34% in patients aged 60 to 69 years (p=0.01) and insignificantly reduced total mortality by 19% in patients aged 30 to 59 years [53-55].

Beta blockers decrease complex VA including VT [55-57]. Beta blockers also increase VF threshold in animal models and have been found to decrease VF in patients with acute MI [58] A randomized, double-blind, placebo-controlled study of propranolol in high-risk survivors of acute MI at 12 Norwegian hospitals showed a 52% significant reduction in sudden cardiac death in patients treated with propranolol for 1 year [58].

Beta blockers decrease myocardial oxygen demand and myocardial ischemia, which may reduce the likelihood of VF. Stone et al [59] showed by 48-hour AECGs in 50 patients with stable angina pectoris that propranolol, but not diltiazem or nifedipine, caused a significant decrease in mean number of episodes of myocardial ischemia and in mean duration of myocardial ischemia compared with placebo. Beta blockers also decrease sympathetic tone, increase vagal tone, and stabilize cardiac membrane potentials which reduces the likelihood of VF. In addition, beta blockers are antithrombotic [60] and may prevent atherosclerotic plaque rupture [61].

In the retrospective study by Hallstrom et al [48] in 941 patients resuscitated from prehospital cardiac arrest attributed to VF, beta blockers were given to 28% of patients and no antiarrhythmic drug to 39% of patients. At 108-month follow-up, patients treated with beta blockers had a significant 38% decreased incidence of death or recurrent cardiac arrest compared to patients treated with no antiarrhythmic [48].

Aronow et al [62] performed a prospective study in 245 persons with heart disease (64% with prior MI and 36% with hypertensive heart disease) and complex VA diagnosed by 24-hour AECGs and a LV ejection fraction ≥40%. Nonsustained VT occurred in 32% of patients. Silent myocardial ischemia occurred in 33% of patients. Of 245 patients, 123 were randomized to propranolol and 122 to no antiarrhythmic drug. Follow-up was 29 months. Propranolol was stopped because of adverse effects in 14 of 123 patients (11%).

Follow-up 24-hour AECGs were obtained at a median of 6 months in 91% of patients treated with propranolol and in 89% of patients treated with no antiarrhythmic drug [62]. Propranolol was significantly more effective than no antiarrhythmic drug in reducing VT >90% (71% versus 25% of patients) and in decreasing the average number of VPCs/hour >70% (71% versus 25% of patients) [62]. The prevalence of silent myocardial ischemia on follow-up 24-hour AECGs was insignificantly higher on no antiarrhythmic drug. However, silent ischemia was significantly abolished by propranolol, with 37% of patients with silent ischemia on their baseline 24-hour AECGs having no silent ischemia on their follow-up 24-hour AECGs [62].

Multivariate Cox regression analyses showed that propranolol caused a 47% significant reduction in sudden cardiac death, a 37% significant decrease in total cardiac death, and a 20% insignificant decrease in total death [62]. Univariate Cox regression analysis showed that among patients taking propranolol, suppression of complex VA caused a 33% insignificant reduction in sudden cardiac death, a 27% insignificant decrease in total cardiac death, and a 30% insignificant reduction in total death [63]. Among patients taking propranolol, abolition of silent myocardial ischemia caused a 70% significant decrease in sudden cardiac death, a 70% significant reduction in total cardiac death, and a 69% significant decrease in total death [63].

There was also a circadian distribution of sudden cardiac death or fatal MI with the peak incidence occurring from 6 AM to 12 PM (peak hour was 8 AM and a secondary peak occurred around 7 PM) in patients treated with no antiarrhythmic drug [64] Propranolol abolished this circadian distribution of sudden cardiac death or fatal MI [64]. In this study, propranolol markedly decreased the circadian variation of complex VA [65] and abolished the circadian variation of myocardial ischemia [66].

In a retrospective analysis of data from the CAST study, Kennedy et al [67] showed that 30% of patients with a LV ejection fraction ≤40% were receiving beta blockers. Patients on beta blockers had a significant decrease in all-cause mortality of 43% at 30 days, of 46% at 1 year, and of 33% at 2 years [67]. Patients treated with beta blockers had a significant reduction in arrhythmic death or cardiac arrest of 66% at 30 days, of 53% at 1 year, and of 36% at 2 years [67]. Multivariate analysis showed that beta blockers were an independent factor for decreasing arrhythmic death or cardiac arrest by 40%, for reducing all-cause mortality by 33%, and for decreasing new or worsened CHF by 32% [67].

ACE inhibitors have been shown to cause a significant reduction in complex VA in patients with CHF in some studies [68, 69] but not in other studies [70, 71]. ACE inhibitors have also been shown to reduce sudden cardiac death in some studies of patients with CHF [32, 72].

ACE inhibitors should be given to reduce total mortality in older and younger patients with CHF [30, 32, 72, 73], an anterior MI [31], an MI with a LV ejection fraction ≤40% [28, 29, 32], and in all patients with atherosclerotic cardiovascular disease [23, 33]. ACE inhibitors should be used to treat patients with CHF with abnormal LV ejection fraction [30, 32, 72, 73] or with normal LV ejection fraction [74, 75].

On the basis of available data, ACE inhibitors should be used to treat patients with VT or complex VA associated with CHF, an anterior MI, an MI with LV systolic dysfunction, or atherosclerotic cardiovascular disease if there are no contraindications to use of ACE inhibitors. Beta blockers should be used in addition to ACE inhibitors in treating these patients.

Class III antiarrhythmic drugs are potassium channel blockers which prolong repolarization manifested by an increase in QT interval on the electrocardiogram. These drugs suppress VA by increasing the refractory period. However, prolonging cardiac repolarization and refractory period can trigger afterdepolarizations and resultant torsade de pointes.

In the Survival With Oral d-Sotalol (SWORD) Trial, 3, 121 survivors of MI with a LV ejection fraction ≤40% were randomized to d-sotalol, a pure potassium channel blocker with no beta blocking activity, or to double-blind placebo [76]. At 148-day follow-up, mortality was 5.0% in patients treated with d-sotalol versus 3.1% in patients treated with placebo [76]. Presumed arrhythmic deaths accounted for the 77% increased mortality (relative risk = 1.77; 95% CI, 1.15 to 2.74) [76].

Studies comparing the effect of d, l-sotalol, a Class III antiarrhythmic drug with beta blocking activity, versus placebo or beta blockers in patients with VT or complex VA have not been performed. In a study of 1, 486 patients with prior MI, compared with placebo, d, l-sotalol did not reduce mortality in patients followed for 1 year [77].

In the Electrophysiologic Study versus Electrocardiographic Monitoring (ESVEM) study of 486 patients, Holter monitor-guided therapy significantly predicted antiarrhythmic drug efficacy more often than did the electrophysiologic study in patients with sustained VT or survivors of cardiac arrest (77% versus 45% of patients) [78]. However, there was no significant difference in the success of drug therapy selected by the two methods in preventing recurrences of ventricular tachyarrhythmias.

In the ESVEM study, d, l-sotalol was more effective than the other 6 antiarrhythmic drugs [imipramine, mexiletine, pirmenol, procainamide, propafenone, and quinidine] used in reducing recurrence of arrhythmia, death from arrhythmia, death from cardiac causes, and death from any cause [79]. However, 7 of 10 episodes of torsade de pointes during this study occurred in patients receiving d, l-sotalol [79]. In 481 patients with VT, d, l-sotalol caused torsade de pointes (12 patients) or an increase in VT episodes (11 patients) in 23 patients (4.9%) [80]. Women had a significantly higher risk for drug-induced VF. On the basis of available data, use of beta blockers is recommended over the use of d, l-sotalol in treating patients with VT or complex VA associated with heart disease.

Amiodarone is very effective in suppressing VT and complex VA associated with heart disease [81-83]. However, the incidence of adverse effects from amiodarone approaches 90% after 5 years of therapy [84]. In the Cardiac Arrest in Seattle: Conventional Versus Amiodarone Drug Evaluation study, the incidence of pulmonary toxicity was 10% at 2 years in patients receiving an amiodarone dose of 158 mg daily [81]. Amiodarone can also cause cardiac adverse effects, gastrointestinal adverse effects including hepatitis, hyperthyroidism, hypothyroidism, and neurologic, dermatologic, and ophthalmologic adverse effects.

A double-blind study randomized 674 patients with CHF and complex VA to amiodarone or placebo [82]. Compared with placebo, amiodarone significantly decreased the number of episodes of VT and the frequency of complex VA. Twenty-seven percent of patients discontinued amiodarone in this study. At 2-year follow-up, survival was not different in patients treated with amiodarone or placebo [82].

The Canadian Amiodarone Myocardial Infarction Arrhythmia Trial (CAMIAT) randomized 1, 202 survivors of MI with nonsustained VT or complex VA to amiodarone or placebo [83] Early permanent discontinuation of amiodarone for reasons other than adverse events occurred in 36% of patients taking this drug [83]. At 1.8-year follow-up, amiodarone caused no significant reduction in mortality [83].

The European Myocardial Infarction Amiodarone Trial (EMIAT) randomized 1, 486 survivors of MI with a LV ejection fraction ≤40% to amiodarone or placebo [85]. Early permanent discontinuation of amiodarone occurred in 38.5% of patients taking this drug. At 21-month follow-up, mortality was similar in patients treated with amiodarone or with placebo [85].

In the Sudden Cardiac Death in Heart Failure Trial (SCD-HEFT), 2, 521 patients with New York Heart Association (NYHA) class II or III CHF due to ischemic or nonischemic heart disease, a LV ejection fraction of 35% or less, and a mean QRS duration on the resting ECG of 120 msec were randomized to placebo, amiodarone, or an automatic implantable cardioverter-defibrillator (AICD) [86]. At 45.5-month median follow-up, compared with placebo, amiodarone insignificantly increased mortality by 6% [86]. At 45.5-month median follow-up, compared with placebo, AICD therapy significantly reduced all-cause mortality by 23%, with an absolute reduction in mortality of 7.2% after 5 years [86].

Since amiodarone has not been found to reduce mortality in patients with VT or complex VA associated with MI or CHF and has a very high incidence of toxicity, beta blockers should be used rather than amiodarone in treating these patients. A meta-analysis of 10 randomized trials showed that the use of beta blockers significantly reduced 2-year mortality in patients receiving AICD therapy [87]. In a study of 965 patients with AICDs, at 32-month mean follow-up, use of beta blockers significantly reduced all-cause mortality by 46%, whereas use of amiodarone or sotalolol did not affect mortality [88]. During 33-month mean follow-up of 1, 038 patients with AICDs, use of beta blockers significantly reduced appropriate AICD shocks [89]. Use of amiodarone plus a beta blocker was not more effective than beta blocker therapy alone in reducing AICD shocks for any reason [89]. In this study, use of sotalol did not reduce appropriate AICD shocks [89].

4. Invasive intervention

If patients have life-threatening recurrent VT or VF resistant to antiarrhythmic drugs, invasive intervention should be performed. Patients with critical coronary artery stenosis and severe myocardial ischemia should undergo coronary artery bypass graft surgery to reduce mortality [90]. In the Coronary Artery Bypass Graft (CABG) Patch Trial, there was no evidence of improved survival among patients with CAD, LV ejection fraction <36%, and an abnormal signal-averaged electrocardiogram undergoing complete coronary revascularization in whom an AICD was implanted prophylactically at the time of elective coronary artery bypass graft surgery [91].

Surgical ablation of the arhythmogenic focus in patients with life-threatening ventricular tachyarrhythmias can be curative. This treatment includes aneurysectomy or infarctectomy and endocardial resection with or without adjunctive cryoablation based on activation mapping in the operating room [92-94]. However, the perioperative mortality rate is high. Endoaneurysmorrhaphy with a pericardial patch combined with mapping-guided subendocardial resection frequently cures recurrent VT with a low operative mortality and improvement of LV systolic function [95]. Radiofrequency catheter ablation of VT has been beneficial in the therapy of selected patients with arrhythmogenic foci of monomorphic VT [96-98]. Catheter ablation has been effectively used to treat patients with right ventricular outflow tract VT and LV fascicular VT. Prophylactic VT ablation should be considered before implantation of an AICD in patients with stable VT, prior MI, and reduced LV ejection fraction [99].

4.1. Automatic implantable cardioverter-defibrillator

However, the AICD is the most effective treatment for patients with life-threatening VT or VF. [93-110]. The Multicenter Automatic Defibrillator Implantation Trial (MADIT) randomized 196 patients, with a prior MI, a LV ejection fraction ≤35%, a documented episode of asymptomatic nonsustained VT, and inducible nonsuppressible ventricular tachyarrhythmia on electrophysiologic study to an AICD or conventional medical therapy [100]. At 27-month follow up, patients receiving an AICD had a 54% significant reduction in mortality [100].

In the Antiarrhythmics versus Implantable Defibrillators (AVID) Trial, 1, 016 patients were randomized to an AICD or class III antiarrhythmic drug therapy [101]. Forty-five percent of patients had been resuscitated from near-fatal VF. The other 55% of patients had sustained VT with syncope or sustained VT with a LV ejection fraction ≤40% and symptoms suggesting severe hemodynamic compromise due to the arrhythmia (near-syncope, CHF, and angina pectoris). The 1-year survival was 89.3% for patients who had the AICD versus 82.3% for patients treated with drug therapy (39% reduction by AICD) [101]. The 2-year survival was 81.6% for patients who had the AICD versus 74.7% for patients treated with drug therapy (27% reduction by AICD) [101]. The 3-year survival was 75.4% for patients who had the AICD versus 64.1% for patients treated with drug therapy (31% reduction by AICD) [101].

The Canadian Implantable Defibrillator Study (CIDS) randomized 659 patients with VF, cardiac arrest, or hypotensive VT to an AICD or amiodarone therapy [102]. Cardiac arrhythmic mortality was 4.5% per year in patients treated with amiodarone versus 3% per year in patients treated with an AICD (risk reduction = 33%). Total mortality was 10.2% per year in patients treated with amiodarone versus 8.3% per year in patients treated with an AICD (risk reduction = 20%) [102]. In a subset of CIDS, at 5.6-year follow-up, 47% of patients treated with amiodarone and 27% of patients treated with an AICD had died [103]. Amiodarone caused adverse effects in 83% of patients receiving the drug [103].

The Cardiac Arrest Study Hamburg (CASH) randomized 230 patients surviving sudden cardiac death due to documented VT and/or VF to propafenone, metoprolol, amiodarone, or an AICD [104]. Propafenone was stopped after 11 months because mortality from sudden death and cardiac arrest recurrence was 23% in patients randomized to propafenone versus 0% in patients randomized to an AICD [104]. The 2-year mortality was 12.6% for 99 patients randomized to an AICD versus 19.6% for 189 patients randomized to amiodarone or metoprolol (37% reduction) [105].

The Multicenter Unsustained Tachycardia Trial randomized 704 patients with inducible, sustained ventricular tachyarrhythmias to 3 treatment groups [106]. Compared with electrophysiologically guided antiarrhythmic drug therapy, the 5-year total mortality was decreased 20% by an AICD, and the 5-year risk of cardiac arrest or death from an arrhythmia was reduced 76% by an AICD [106]. Neither total mortality incidence or rate of cardiac arrest or death from arrhythmia was lower in patients randomized to electrophysiologically guided therapy and treated with antiarrhythmic drugs than in patients randomized to no antiarrhythmic treatment [106].

MADIT II randomized 1, 232 patients with prior MI and a LV ejection fraction of ≤30% to an AICD or to conventional medical therapy [107]. At 20-month follow-up, compared with conventional medical therapy, the AICD reduced all-cause mortality 31% from 19.8% to 14.2% [107]. The effect of AICD therapy in improving survival was similar in patients stratified according to age, sex, LV ejection fraction, New York Heart Association class, and QRS interval [107].

In MADIT-II, the reduction in sudden cardiac death in patients treated with an AICD was significantly reduced by 68% in 574 patients aged <65 years, by 65% in 455 patients aged 65-74 years, and by 68% in 204 patients aged ≥75 years [108]. The median survival in 348 octogenarians treated with AICD therapy was >4years [109].

At 8-year follow-up in MADIT II, the cumulative probability of all-cause mortality was 49% for patients treated with an AICD versus 62% for patients not treated with an AICD [110]. AICD treatment caused a 34% reduction in mortality during treatment years 1-4 and a 26% reduction in mortality during years 5-8 [110].

After AICD implantation, 35 patients were randomized to treatment with metoprolol and 35 patients to treatment with d, l-sotalol [111]. VT recurrence was 17% at 1 year and 20% at 2 years for patients treated with metoprolol versus 43% at 1 year and 49% at 2 years for patients treated with d, l-sotalol. At 26-month follow-up, survival was 91% for patients treated with metoprolol plus an AICD versus 83% for patients treated with d, l-sotalol plus an AICD [111]. In MADIT-II, use of higher doses of beta blockers in patients with ischemic heart disease and an AICD significantly reduced mortality by 56-58% compared with non-use of beta blockers [112]. These data favor using a beta blocker in patients with an AICD.

At 32-month mean follow-up of 965 patients, death occurred in 73 of 515 patients (13%) treated with beta blockers, in 84 of 494 patients (17%) treated with ACE inhibitors or angiotensin receptor blockers, in 56 of 402 patients (14%) treated with statins, in 40 of 227 patients (18%) treated with amiodarone, in 5 of 26 patients (19%) treated with sotalol, and in 64 of 265 patients (24%) treated with no beta blocker, ACE inhibitor, angiotensin receptor blocker, statin, amiodarone, or sotalol [88]. These data favor treating patients with AICDs with beta blockers, statins, and ACE inhibitors or angiotensin receptor blockers.

The American College of Cardiology Foundation (ACCF)/American Heart Association (AHA) guidelines(Table 1) recommend that Class I indications for therapy with an AICD are 1) cardiac arrest due to VF or VT not due to a transient or a reversible cause; 2) spontaneous sustained VT; 3) syncope of undetermined origin with clinically relevant, hemodynamically significant sustained VT or VF induced at electrophysiologic study when drug therapy is ineffective, not tolerated, or not preferred; ; 4) patients with prior MI at least 40 days previously with a LV ejection fraction less than 35% who are in NYHA class II or III; 5) patients with nonischemic dilated cardiomyopathy with a LV ejection fraction less than or equal to 35% who are in NYHA class II or III; 6) patients with prior MI at least 40 days previously with a LV ejection fraction less than 30% who are in NYHA class I; and 7) patients with nonsustained VT due to prior MI with a LV ejection fraction less than 40% and inducible VF or sustained VT at electrophysiological study [113].

1. Survivors of cardiac arrest due to VF or hemodynamically unstable sustained VT after evaluation to diagnose the cause and to exclude completely reversible causes
2. Structural heart disease and spontaneous sustained VT, whether hemodynamically stable or unstable
3. Syncope of undetermined etiology with clinically relevant, hemodynamically significant sustained VT or VF induced at electrophysiological study
4. LV ejection fraction less than 35% due to prior MI at least 40 days previously and NYHA class II or III
5. Nonischemic dilated cardiomyopathy with LV ejection fraction less than or equal to 35% and NYHA class II or III
6. LV ejection fraction less than 30% due to prior myocardial infarction at least 40 days previously and NYHA class I
7. Nonsustained VT due to MI, LV ejection fraction less than 40%, and inducible VF or sustained VT at electrophysiological study

Table 1. Class I indications for Automatic Implantable Cardioverter-Defibrillator

Adapted from Epstein AE et al [113]

The 2009 updated ACCF/AHA guidelines for treatment of CHF (Table 2) recommend with a class I indication use of an AICD for 1) secondary prevention to increase survival in patients with current or prior symptoms of heart failure and decreased LV ejection fraction who have a history of cardiac arrest, VF, or hemodynamically destabilizing VT; 2) primary prevention of sudden cardiac death to reduce mortality in patients with nonischemic dilated cardiomyopathy or CAD at least 40 days after MI, a LV ejection fraction less than or equal to 35%, and NYHA class II or III symptoms on optimal medical therapy, with expectation of survival with good functional status for more than 1 year; and 3) may be used in patients receiving cardiac resynchronization therapy (CRT) for NYHA class III or ambulatory class IV symptoms despite recommended optimal medical therapy [114, 115].

1. Secondary prevention to increase survival in patients with current or prior symptoms of heart failure and reduced LV ejection fraction with a history of cardiac arrest, VF, or hemodynamically destabilizing VT
2. Primary prevention of sudden cardiac death to reduce mortality in patients with nonischemic dilated cardiomyopathy or ischemic heart disease at least 40 days after MI, a LV ejection fraction less than or equal to 35%, and NYHA class II or III symptoms on optimal medical therapy, with expectation of survival with good functional status for more than 1 year
3. May be used in patients receiving cardiac resynchronization therapy for NYHA class III or ambulatory class IV symptoms despite recommended optimal medical therapy

Table 2. Class I Indications for Implantation of an Automatic Implantable Cardioverter-Defibrillator in Congestive Heart Failure

Adapted from Jessup M et al [114]

The ACC/AHA guidelines class IIa indications for treatment with an AICD are listed in Table 3 [113].

1. Unexplained syncope, significant LV dysfunction, and nonischemic dilated cardiomyopathy
2. Sustained VT and normal or near normal LV function
3. Hypertrophic cardiomyopathy with 1 or more major risk factor for SCD
4. Prevention of SCD in patients with arrhythmogenic right ventricular dysplasia/cardiomyopathy who have 1 or more risk factor for SCD
5. Reduction of SCD in patients with long-QT syndrome who are having syncope and/or VT while using beta blockers
6. Nonhospitalized patients awaiting cardiac transplantation
7. Brugada syndrome with syncope
8. Brugada syndrome with documented VT that has not resulted in cardiac arrest
9. Catecholaminergic polymorphic VT with syncope and/or documented sustained VT while using beta blockers
10. Cardiac sarcoidosis, giant cell myocarditis, or Chagas disease

Table 3. Class IIa Indications for Implantation of an Automatic Implantable Cardioverter-Defibrillator

Adapted from Epstein AE et al [113]

If the patient has no indication for pacing and a normal LV ejection fraction, CRT should not be performed. If the patient has no indication for pacing and a reduced LV ejection fraction, CRT should not be performed

An AICD may also be effective in preventing sudden death in patients with hypertrophic cardiomyopathy at high risk for sudden death [116] and in patients at high risk for sudden death because of a long QT interval or the Brugada syndrome [117]. An AICD may be useful in preventing sudden death in patients with syncope and ventricular tachyarrhythmias associated with poor LV ejection fraction, regardless of the result of the electrophysiologic study [118]. In addition, an AICD may be useful in survivors of VT or VF as a bridge to cardiac transplantation [119].

AICDs were implanted in 378 men and 95 women [120]. At 3.6-year follow-up, survival was 76% in patients who had an AICD because of cardiac arrest due to VF or VT not due to a transient or reversible cause, 85% in patients who had an AICD because of spontaneous sustained VT in association with structural heart disease, 92% in patients who had an AICD because of syncope of undetermined origin with clinically relevant, hemodynamically sustained VT or VF induced at electrophysiological study when drug therapy is ineffective, not tolerated, or not preferred, 84% in patients who had an AICD because of nonsustained VT with CAD, MI, LV dysfunction, and inducible VF or sustained VT at electrophysiological study that is not suppressible by a Class I antiarrhythmic drug, and 85% in all 473 patients [120].

AICDs are not effective in treating patients with LV dysfunction scheduled for elective CABG [91] or in patients who have had an acute MI within 40 days of the procedure [121, 122]. In patients receiving AICDs early after MI, factors associated with arrhythmias needing AICD therapy are also associated with a high risk of nonsudden death, negating the benefit of AICDs [123]. AICDs should also not be used to treat patients with NYHA class IV CHF despite optimal medical management or in patients with a life expectancy less than 1 year [114]

Of 209 patients with NYHA class III or IV heart failure treated with combined CRT-AICD therapy, appropriate cardioverter-defibrillator shocks occurred at 34-month follow-up in 22 of 121 patients (18%) on statins and in 30 of 88 patients (34%) not on statins [124]. Death occurred in 3 of 121 patients (2%) on statins and in 9 of 88 patients (10%) not on statins. Stepwise Cox regression analysis showed that significant independent prognostic factors for appropriate shocks were use of statins (risk ratio = 0.46), smoking (risk ratio = 3.5); and diabetes mellitus (risk ratio = 0.34) [124]. Significant independent prognostic factors for the time to mortality were use of statins (risk ratio = 0.05), use of digoxin (risk ratio = 4.2), hypertension (risk ratio = 14.2), diabetes mellitus (risk ratio = 4.3), and LV ejection fraction (risk ratio = 1.1) [124].

Of 529 patients with CHF and a reduced LV ejection fraction, 209 (40%) were treated with CRT plus an AICD and 320 (60%) with an AICD [125]. Mean follow-up was 34 months for both groups. Stepwise logistic regression analysis showed that significant independent variables for appropriate AICD shocks were statins (risk ratio = 0.35), smoking (risk ratio = 2.52), and digoxin (risk ratio = 1.92). Significant independent variables for time to deaths were use of CRT (risk ratio = 0.32), statins (risk ratio = 0.18), ACE inhibitors/angiotensin receptor blockers (ARBs) (risk ratio = 0.10), hypertension (risk ratio = 24.15), diabetes (risk ratio = 2.54), and age (risk ratio = 1.06) [125].

During 1243 days mean follow-up of 549 patients who had an AICD for CHF, 163 (30%) had appropriate AICD shocks, 71 (13%) had inappropriate AICD shocks, and 63 (12%) died [126]. Stepwise logistic regression analysis showed that significant independent prognostic factors for appropriate AICD shocks were smoking (odds ratio = 3.7) and statins (odds ratio = 0.54), for inappropriate AICD shocks were atrial fibrillation (odds ratio = 6.2) and statins (odds ratio = 0.52), and for time to mortality were age (hazard ratio = 1.08 per 1-year increase), ACE inhibitors or angiotensin receptor blockers ARBs (hazard ratio = 0.25), atrial fibrillation (hazard ratio = 4.1), right ventricular pacing (hazard ratio = 3.6), digoxin (hazard ratio = 2.9), hypertension (hazard ratio = 5.3), and statins (hazard ratio = 0.32) [126].

AICDs were implanted in 485 patients with ischemic cardiomyopathy and in 299 patients with nonischemic cardiomyopathy [127]. At 33-month follow-up, appropriate ICD shocks occurred in 179 of 485 patients (37%) with ischemic cardiomyopathy and in 93 of 299 patients (31%) with nonischemic cardiomyopathy. All-cause mortality occurred in 162 of 485 patients (33%) with ischemic cardiomyopathy and in 70 of 299 patients (23%) with nonischemic cardiomyopathy [127].

During implantatation and during 38-month follow-up of 1, 060 patients who had AICDs, complications occurred in 60 patients (5.7%) [128]. These complications consisted of fractured leads requiring lead revision in 36 patients (3.4%), lead infection requiring antibiotics in 5 patients (0.5%), device replacement because of malfunction in 5 patients (0.5%), repositioning of leads in 3 patients (0.3%), a hematoma at the time of implantation in 3 patients (0.3%), pneumothorax at the time of implantation in 2 patients (0.2%), repair of a defective generator in 1 patient (0.1%), replacement of the device because of atrophy of the skin over the device in 1 patient (0.1%), a transient ischemic attack because of atrial fibrillation developing during implantation in 1 patient (0.1%), device replacement because of a recall from Guidant in 1 patient (0.1%), pocket revision because of pain when lying on the side of the pacemaker in 1 patient (0.1%), and pacemaker infection in 1 patient (0.1%) [128]. A downloadable algorithm has been developed to reduce inappropriate shocks caused by fractures of implantable AICD leads [129].

Persistent atrial fibrillation is associated with appropriate shocks and with CHF in patients with LV dysfunction treated with an AICD [130]. One or more inappropriate AICD shocks occurred in 83 of 719 MADIT II patients (11.5%) and comprised 31.2% of 590 shocks [131]. Triggers for inappropriate shocks were atrial fibrillation (44%), supraventricular tachycardia (36%), and abnormal sensing (20%). Patients with inappropriate shocks had a 2.3 times increase in mortality [131].

In 1, 193 patients with combined CRT-AICD therapy, atrial tachycardia/atrial fibrillation lasting longer than 10 minutes occurred in 361 patients (30%) [132]. Device-detected atrial tachycardia/atrial fibrillation was associated with a 2.16 times increased mortality at 13 months median follow-up [132].

Of 958 patients with an AICD, chronic kidney disease was a significant independent predictor of 1-year mortality [133]. The 1-year mortality was 1.8%, 5.3%, 9.0%, 22%, and 38% for stages 1, 2, 3, 4, and 5, respectively of renal function. [133].

Successful radiofrequecy ablation was performed in 22 of 84 patients with an AICD who had inappropriate shocks from atrial tachycardia, atrial flutter, or atrioventricular nodal reentrant tachycardia [134]. Ninety-five percent of 22 patients who underwent successful radiofrequency ablation for supraventricular tachycardia had no inappropriate AICD shocks at 21-month follow-up compared to 63% of patients with inappropriate shocks for supraventricular tachycardia who did not have radiofrequency ablation [134].

In patients with AICDs, compared to patients treated with ventricular backup pacing at a rate of 40/minute, patients treated with dual-chamber rate-responsive pacing at a rate of 70/minute (DDDR-70) had an increase in mortality [135, 136], worsening of LV ejection fraction [137], and an increase in new LV wall motion abnormality [137]. One reason why DDDR-70 pacing may increase mortality and worsen LV systolic function is that ventricular electrical activation proceeds from the right ventricular apex instead of through the existing conduction system.

In patients with AICDs and no indication for antibradycardia pacing, 22 of 80 patients (28%) treated with right ventricular pacing died at 45-month follow-up, and 8 of 81 patients (10%) treated with biventricular pacing died at 53-month follow-up [138]. At 23-month follow-up, the LV ejection fraction decreased from 36% to 30% in patients treated with right ventricular pacing and increased at 38-month follow-up from 35% to 40% in patients treated with biventricular pacing [138]. New LV wall motion abnormality developed at 23-month follow-up in 23 of 80 patients (29%) treated with right ventricular pacing and at 38-month follow-up in 7 of 81 patients (9%) treated with biventricular pacing [138]. On the basis of available data, patients with AICDs should be treated with biventricular pacing, not with DDDR-70 right ventricular pacing [135-138].

In the Multicenter Automatic Defibrillator Implantation Trial with Cardiac Resynchronization Therapy (MADIT-CRT) trial of 821 patients with nonischemic cardiomyopatyhy, 499 (61%) were treated with statins [139]. At 4-year follow-up, the cumulative probability of fast VT/VF or death was significantly reduced in patients treated with statins (11%) than in patients not treated with statins (19%) [139].

In the 1, 1820 patients in the MADIT-CRT trial, CRT -defibrillator therapy reduced first ventricular tachyarrhythmic events by 42% in patients with a left bundle branch block but did not reduce first ventricular tachyarrhythmic events in patients without left bundle branch block [140]. Recurrent ventricular tachyarrhythmic events were not reduced in patients with a left bundle branch block and were increased 3.62 times in patients without a left bundle branch block [140].

At 1.4-year follow-up of 1, 500 patients treated with an AICD for primary prevention, compared with conventional programming, programming the AICD for tachyarrhythmias of

200 beats per minute or higher was associated with a significant 79% reduction in inappropriate shocks or inappropriate antitachycardia pacing and a significant 55% reduction in all-cause mortality [141]. Compared with conventional programming, a prolonged delay in AICD therapy to 170 beats per minute or higher was associated with a significant 76% reduction in inappropriate shocks or inappropriate antitachycardia pacing and a significant 44% reduction in all-cause mortality [141].

At 1-year follow-up of 1, 902 patients treated with an AICD for primary or secondary prevention, use of a long-versus standard-detection interval caused a 42% significant reduction in antitachycardia pacing, a 23% insignificant reduction in appropriate shocks, a 45% significant reduction in inappropriate shocks, and a 13% insignificant reduction in mortality [142].

In a registry of 5, 399 AICD recipients for primary and secondary prevention, rates of appropriate shocks were similar among patients aged 18-49, 50-59, 60-69, 70-79, and ≥ 80 years [143]. There was no significant difference in mortality between clinical trial patients randomized to an AICD for primary prevention in the MADIT-II and SCD-HEFT trials and a similar group of clinical registry patient who received an AICD for primary prevention [144].

In patients with an AICD and a CRT-defibrillator, 3, 809 patients who survived a first shock were matched to 3, 630 patients without a shock [145]. Compared with no shock, mortality was significantly increased 1.65 times in those who received a shock for monomorphic VT, 2.1 times for those who received a shock for VF/polymorphic VT, and 161 times for those who received a shock for atrial fibrillation/atrial flutter [145]. Mortality was similar in those who received a shock for sinus tachycardia, supraventricular tachycardia, and noise/artefact oversensing compared to no shock [145].

Author details

Wilbert S. Aronow*

Cardiology Division, Department of Medicine, Westchester Medical Center/New York Medical College, Valhalla, NY, USA

The author has no conflicts of interest.

References

[1] Fleg JL, Kennedy HL. Cardiac arrhythmia in a healthy elderly population. Detection by 24-hour ambulatory electrocardiography. Chest 1982;81:302-307.

[2] Aronow WS, Mercando AD, Epstein S. Prevalence of arrhythmias detected by 24-hour ambulatory electrocardiography and the value of antiarrhythmic therapy in elderly patients with unexplained syncope. Am J Cardiol 1992;70:408-410.

[3] Aronow WS, Epstein S, Mercando AD. Usefulness of complex ventricular arrhythmias detected by 24-hour ambulatory electrocardiogram and by electrocardiograms with one-minute rhythm strips in predicting new coronary events in elderly patients with and without heart disease. J Cardiovasc Technol 1991;10:21-25.

[4] Camm AJ, Evans KE, Ward DE, Martin A. The rhythm of the heart in active elderly subjects. Am Heart J 1980;99:598-603.

[5] Kantelip JP, Sage E, Duchene-Marullaz P. Findings on ambulatory electrocardiographic monitoring in subjects older than 80 years. Am J Cardiol 1986;57:398-401.

[6] Manolio TA, Furberg CD, Rautaharju PM, et al. Cardiac arrhythmias on 24-h ambulatory electrocardiography in older women and men: The Cardiovascular Health Study. J Am Coll Cardiol 1994;23:916-925.

[7] Aronow WS, Ahn C, Mercando A, et al. Prevalence and association of ventricular tachycardia and complex ventricular arrhythmias with new coronary events in older men and women with and without cardiovascular disease. J Gerontol: Med Sci 2002;57A:M178-M180.

[8] Aronow WS, Epstein S, Schwartz KS, Koenigsberg M. Prevalence of arrhythmias detected by ambulatory electrocardiographic monitoring and of abnormal left ventricular ejection fraction in persons older than 62 years in a long-term health care facility. Am J Cardiol 1987;59;368-369.

[9] Aronow WS, Epstein S, Schwartz KS, Koenigsberg M. Correlation of complex ventricular arrhythmias detected by ambulatory electrocardiographic monitoring with echocardiographic left ventricular hypertrophy in persons older than 62 years in a long-term health care facility. Am J Cardiol 1987;60:730-732.

[10] Aronow WS, Epstein S. Usefulness of silent ischemia, ventricular tachycardia, and complex ventricular arrhythmias in predicting new coronary events in elderly patients with coronary artery disease or systemic hypertension. Am J Cardiol 1990;65:511-522.

[11] Fleg JL, Kennedy HL. Long-term prognostic significance of ambulatory electrocardiographic findings in apparently healthy subjects ≥60 years of age. Am J Cardiol 1992;70:748-751.

[12] Fleg JL, Lakatta EG. Prevalence and prognosis of exercise-induced nonsustained ventricular tachycardia in apparently healthy volunteers. Am J Cardiol 1984;54:762-764.

[13] Busby MJ, Shefrin EA, Fleg JL. Prevalence and long-term significance of exercise-induced frequent or repetitive ventricular ectopic beats in apparently healthy volunteers. J Am Coll Cardiol 1989;14:1659-1665.

[14] Aronow WS, Epstein S, Koenigsberg M, Schwartz KS. Usefulness of echocardiographic abnormal left ventricular ejection fraction, paroxysmal ventricular tachycar-

dia, and complex ventricular arrhythmias in predicting new coronary events in patients over 62 years of age. Am J Cardiol 1988;61:1349-1351.

[15] Aronow WS, Epstein S, Koenigsberg M, Schwartz KS. Usefulness of echocardiographic left ventricular hypertrophy, ventricular tachycardia and complex ventricular arrhythmias in predicting ventricular fibrillation or sudden cardiac death in elderly patients. Am J Cardiol 1988;62:1124-1125.

[16] Moss AJ, Davis HT, DeCamilla J, Bayer LW. Ventricular ectopic beats and their relation to sudden and nonsudden death after myocardial infarction. Circulation 1979;60:998-1003.

[17] Bigger JT, Fleiss JL, Kleiger R, et al. The relationships among ventricular arrhythmias, left ventricular dysfunction, and mortality in the 2 years after myocardial infarction. Circulation 1984;69:250-258.

[18] Mukharji J, Rude RE, Poole WK, et al. Risk factors for sudden death after acute myocardial infarction: Two-year follow-up. Am J Cardiol 1984;54:31-36.

[19] Kostis JB, Byington R, Friedman LM, et al. Prognostic significance of ventricular ectopic activity in survivors of acute myocardial infarction. J Am Coll Cardiol 1987;10:231-242.

[20] Antithrombotic Trialists' Collaboration. Collaborative meta-analysis of randomised trials of antiplatelet therapy for prevention of death, myocardial infarction, and stroke in high risk patients. Br Med J 2002;324:71-86.

[21] Goldstein RE, Andrews M, Hall WJ, et al. Marked reduction in long-term cardiac deaths with aspirin after a coronary event. J Am Coll Cardiol 1996;28:326-330.

[22] Aronow WS, Ahn C. Reduction of coronary events with aspirin in older patients with prior myocardial infarction treated with and without statins. Heart Dis 2002;4:159-161.

[23] Smith SC Jr, Benjamin EJ,, Bonow RO, et al. AHA/ACCF secondary prevention and risk reduction therapy for patients with coronary and other atherosclerotic cardiovascular disease: 2011 update. A guideline from the American Heart Association and American College of Cardiology Foundation. J Am Coll Cardiol 2011; 58:2432-2446.

[24] Hjalmarson A, Elmfeldt D, Herlitz J, et al. Effect on mortality of metoprolol in acute myocardial infarction. Lancet 1981;2:823-827.

[25] Gundersen T, Abrahamsen AM, Kjekshus J, et al. Timolol-related reduction in mortality and reinfarction in patients ages 65-75 years surviving acute myocardial infarction. Circulation 1982; 66:1179-1184.

[26] Pedersen TR for the Norwegian Multicentre Study Group. Six-year follow-up of the Norwegian Multicentre Study on Timolol after acute myocardial infarction. N Engl J Med 1985;313:1055-1058.

[27] Beta-Blocker Heart Attack Trial Research Group. A randomized trial of propranolol in patients with acute myocardial infarction. JAMA 1982; 247:1707-1714.

[28] Aronow WS, Ahn C, Kronzon I. Effect of beta blockers alone, of angiotensin-converting enzyme inhibitors alone, and of beta blockers plus angiotensin-converting enzyme inhibitors on new coronary events and on congestive heart failure in older persons with healed myocardial infarcts and asymptomatic left ventricular systolic dysfunction. Am J Cardiol 2001;88:1298-1300.

[29] Pfeffer MA, Braunwald E, Moye LA, et al. Effect of captopril on mortality and morbidity in patients with left ventricular dysfunction after myocardial infarction. Results of the Survival and Ventricular Enlargement Trial. N Engl J Med 1992;327:669-677.

[30] The Acute Infarction Ramipril Efficacy (AIRE) Study Investigators. Effect of ramipril on mortality and morbidity of survivors of acute myocardial infarction with clinical evidence of heart failure. Lancet 1993;342:821-828.

[31] Ambrosioni E, Borghi C, Magnani B, for the Survival of Myocardial Infarction Long-Term Evaluation (SMILE) Study Investigators. The effect of the angiotensin-converting-enzyme inhibitor zofenopril on mortality and morbidity after anterior myocardial infarction. N Engl J Med 1995;332:80-85.

[32] Kober L, Torp-Pedersen C, Carlsen JE, et al. A clinical trial of the angiotensin-converting-enzyme inhibitor trandolapril in patients with left ventricular dysfunction after myocardial infarction. N Engl J Med 1995;333:1670-1676.

[33] HOPE (Heart Outcomes Prevention Evaluation) Study Investigators. Effects of an angiotensin-converting-enzyme inhibitor, ramipril, on cardiovascular events in high-risk patients. N Engl J Med 2000;342:145-153.

[34] Miettinen TA, Pyorala K, Olsson AG, et al. Cholesterol-lowering therapy in women and elderly patients with myocardial infarction or angina pectoris. Findings from the Scandinavian Simvastatin Survival Study (4S). Circulation 1997;96:4211-4218.

[35] Lewis SJ, Moye LA, Sacks FM, et al. Effect of pravastatin on cardiovascular events in older patients with myocardial infarction and cholesterol levels in the average range. Results of the Cholesterol and Recurrent Events (CARE) Trial. Ann Intern Med 1998;129:681-689.

[36] The Long-Term Intervention with Pravastatin in Ischaemic Disease (LIPID) Study Group. Prevention of cardiovascular events and death with pravastatin in patients with coronary heart disease and a broad range of initial cholesterol levels. N Engl J Med 1998;339:1349-1357.

[37] Aronow WS, Ahn C. Incidence of new coronary events in older persons with prior myocardial infarction and serum low-density lipoprotein cholesterol ≥125 mg/dL treated with statins versus no lipid-lowering drug. Am J Cardiol. 2002;89:67-69.

[38] Heart Protection Study Collaborative Group. MRC/BHF Heart Protection Study of cholesterol lowering with simvastatin in 20, 536 high-risk individuals: a randomised placebo-controlled trial. Lancet. 2002;360:7-22.

[39] Shepherd J, Blauw GJ, Murphy MB, et al. Pravastatin in elderly individuals at risk of vascular disease (PROSPER): a randomised controlled trial. Lancet 2002:360:1623-1630.

[40] Stone NJ, Robinson J, Lichtenstein AH, et al. ACC/AHA guideline on the treatment of blood cholesterol to reduce atherosclerotic cardiovascular risk in adults. A Report of the American College of Cardiology/American Heart Association Task Force on Practice Guidelines. Endorsed by the American Association of Cardiovascular and Pulmonary Rehabilitation, American Pharmacists Association, American Society for Preventive Cardiology, Association of Black Cardiologists, Preventive Cardiovascular Nurses Association, and WomenHeart: The National Coalition for Women with Heart Disease. J Am Coll Cardiol 2013; published online November 12, 2013.

[41] Frishman WH Aronow WS, Cheng-Lai A. Cardiovascular drug therapy in the elderly. In: Aronow WS, Fleg J, Rich MW, eds. Cardiovascular Disease in the Elderly, fourth edition, New York City: Informa Healthcare 2008:99-135

[42] IMPACT Research Group. International Mexiletine and Placebo Antiarrhythmic Coronary Trial: I. Report on arrhythmia and other findings. J Am Coll Cardiol 1984;4:1148-1163

[43] The Cardiac Arrhythmia Suppression Trial (CAST) Investigators. Preliminary report. Effect of encainide and flecainide on mortality in a randomized trial of arrhythmia suppression after myocardial infarction. N Engl J Med 1989;321:406-412.

[44] Akiyama T, Pawitan Y, Campbell WB, et al. Effects of advancing age on the efficacy and side effects of antiarrhythmic drugs in post-myocardial infarction patients with ventricular arrhythmias. J Am Geriatr Soc 1992;40:666-672.

[45] The Cardiac Arrhythmia Suppression Trial II Investigators. Effect of the antiarrhythmic agent moricizine on survival after myocardial infarction. N Engl J Med 1992;327:227-233.

[46] Aronow WS, Mercando AD, Epstein S, Kronzon I. Effect of quinidine or procainamide versus no antiarrhythmic drug on sudden cardiac death, total cardiac death, and total death in elderly patients with heart disease and complex ventricular arrhythmias. Am J. Cardiol 1990;66:423-428.

[47] Moosvi AR, Goldstein S, VanderBrug Medendorp S, et al. Effect of empiric antiarrhythmic therapy in resuscitated out-of-hospital cardiac arrest victims with coronary artery disease. Am J Cardiol 1990;65:1192-1197.

[48] Hallstrom AP, Cobb LA, Hui Yu B, et al. An antiarrhythmic drug experience in 941 patients resuscitated from an initial cardiac arrest between 1970 and 1985. Am J Cardiol 1991;68:1025-1031.

[49] Coplen SE, Antmann EM, Berlin JA, et al. Efficacy and safety of quinidine therapy for maintenance of sinus rhythm after cardioversion: A meta-analysis of randomized control trials. Circulation 1990;82:1106-1116.

[50] Flaker GC, Blackshear JL, McBride R, et al. Antiarrhythmic drug therapy and cardiac mortality in atrial fibrillation. J Am Coll Cardiol 1992;20:527-532.

[51] Morganroth J, Goin JE. Quinidine-related mortalitiy in the short-to-medium term treatment of ventricular arrhythmias. A meta-analysis. Circulation 1991;84:1977-1983.

[52] Teo KK, Yusuf S, Furberg CD. Effects of prophylactic antiarrhythmic drug therapy in acute myocardial infarction. An overview of results from randomized controlled trials. JAMA 1993;270:1589-1595.

[53] Hawkins CM, Richardson DW, Vokonas PS, for the BHAT Research Group. Effect of propranolol in reducing mortality in older myocardial infarction patients. The Beta-Blocker Heart Attack Trial experience. Circulation 1983;67[suppl I]:I-94-I-97.

[54] Friedman LM, Byington RP, Capone RJ, et al. Effect of propranolol in patients with myocardial infarction and ventricular arrhythmia. J Am Coll Cardiol 1986;7:1-8.

[55] Lichstein E, Morganroth J, Harrist R, et al. Effect of propranolol on ventricular arrhythmia. The Beta-Blocker Heart Attack Trial experience. Circulation 1983;67[suppl I]:I-5-I-10.

[56] Hansteen V. Beta blockade after myocardial infarction: The Norwegian Propranolol Study in high-risk patients. Circulation 1983;67[suppl I]:I-57-I-60.

[57] de Soyza N, Shapiro W, Chandraratna PAN, et al. Acebutolol for ventricular arrythmia: A randomized, placebo-controlled, double-blind multicenter study. Circulation 1982;65:1129-1133.

[58] Norris RM, Barnaby PF, Brown MA, et al. Prevention of ventricular fibrillation during acute myocardial infarction by intravenous propranolol. Lancet 1984;2:883-886.

[59] Stone PH, Gibson RS, Glasser SP, et al. Comparison of propranolol, diltiazem, and nifedipine in the treatment of ambulatory ischemia in patients with stable angina. Differential effects on ambulatory ischemia, exercise performance, and anginal symptoms. Circulation 1990;82:1962-1972.

[60] Weksler BB, Gillick M, Pink J. Effects of propranolol on platelet function. Blood 1977;49:185-196.

[61] Frishman WH, Lazar EJ. Reduction of mortality, sudden death and non-fatal infarction with beta-adrenergic blockers in survivors of acute myocardial infarction: A new

hypothesis regarding the cardioprotective action of beta-adrenergic blockade. Am J Cardiol 1990;66(suppl):66G-70G.

[62] Aronow WS, Ahn C, Mercando AD, et al. Effect of propranolol versus no antiarrhythmic drug on sudden cardiac death, total cardiac death, and total death in patients ≥62 years of age with heart disease, complex ventricular arrhythmias, and left ventricular ejection fraction ≥40%. Am J Cardiol 1994;74:267-270.

[63] Aronow WS, Ahn C, Mercando AD, et al. Decrease of mortality by propranolol in patients with heart disease and complex ventricular arrhythmias is more an anti-ischemic than an antiarrhythmic effect. Am J Cardiol 1994;74:613-615.

[64] Aronow WS, Ahn C, Mercando AD, Epstein S. Circadian variation of sudden cardiac death or fatal myocardial infarction is abolished by propranolol in patients with heart disease and complex ventricular arrhythmias. Am J Cardiol 1994;74:819-821.

[65] Aronow WS, Ahn C, Mercando AD, Epstein S. Effect of propranolol on circadian variation of ventricular arrhythmias in elderly patients with heart disease and complex ventricular arrhythmias. Am J Cardiol 1995;75:514-516.

[66] Aronow WS, Ahn C, Mercando AD, Epstein S. Effect of propranolol on circadian variation of myocardial ischemia in elderly patients with heart disease and complex ventricular arrhythmias. Am J Cardiol 1995;75:837-839.

[67] Kennedy HL, Brooks MM, Barker AH, et al. Beta-blocker therapy in the Cardiac Arrhythmia Suppression Trial. Am J Cardiol 1994;74:674-680.

[68] Webster MW, Fitzpatrick MA, Nicholls MG, et al. Effect of enalapril on ventricular arrhythmias in congestive heart failure. Am J Cardiol 1985;56:566-569.

[69] Fletcher RD, Cintron GB, Johnson G, et al. Enalapril decreases prevalence of ventricular tachycardia in patients with chronic congestive heart failure. Circulation 1993;87[suppl VI]:VI-49-VI-55.

[70] Pratt CM, Gardner M, Pepine C, et al. Lack of long-term ventricular arrhythmia reduction by enalapril in heart failure. Am J Cardiol 1995;75:1244-1249.

[71] Aronow WS, Mercando AD, Epstein S. Effect of benazepril on complex ventricular arrhythmias in older patients with congestive heart failure, prior myocardial infarction, and normal left ventricular ejection fraction. Am J Cardiol 1998;81:1368-1370.

[72] Cohn JN, Johnson G, Ziesche S, et al. A comparison of enalapril with hydralazine-isosorbide dinitrate in the treatment of chronic congestive heart failure. N Engl J Med 1991;325:303-310.

[73] Garg R, Yusuf S, for the Collaborative Group on ACE Inhibitor Trials. Overview of randomized trials of angiotensin-converting enzyme inhibitors on mortality and morbidity in patients with heart failure. JAMA 1995;273:1450-1456.

[74] Aronow WS, Kronzon I. Effect of enalapril on congestive heart failure treated with diuretics in elderly patients with prior myocardial infarction and normal left ventricular ejection fraction. Am J Cardiol 1993;71:602-604.

[75] Philbin EF, Rocco TA Jr, Lindenmuth NW, et al. Systolic versus diastolic heart failure in community practice: clinical features, outcomes, and the use of angiotensin-converting enzyme inhibitors. Am J Med 2000;109:605-613.

[76] Waldo AL, Camm AJ, deRuyter H, et al. Effect of d-sotalol on mortality in patients with left ventricular dysfunction after recent and remote myocardial infarction. Lancet 1996;348:7-12.

[77] Julian DJ, Prescott RJ, Jackson FS, Szekely P. Controlled trial of sotalol for one year after myocardial infarction. Lancet 1982;1:1142-1147.

[78] Mason JW for the Electrophysiologic Study versus Electrocardiographic Monitoring Investigators. A comparison of electrophysiologic testing with Holter monitoring to predict antiarrhythmic-drug efficacy for ventricular tachyarrhythmias. N Engl J Med 1993;329:445-451.

[79] Mason JW for the Electrophysiologic Study versus Electrocardiographic Monitoring Investigators. A comparison of seven antiarrhythmic drugs in patients with ventricular tachyarrhythmias. N Engl J Med 1993;329:452-458.

[80] Kehoe RF, MacNeil DJ, Zheutlin TA, et al. Safety and efficacy of oral sotalol for sustained ventricular tachyarrhythmias refractory to other antiarrhythmic agents. Am J Cardiol 1993;72:56A-66A.

[81] Greene HL for the CASCADE Investigators. The CASCADE study. Randomized antiarrhythmic drug therapy in survivors of cardiac arrest in Seattle. Am J Cardiol 1993;72:70F-74F.

[82] Singh SN, Fletcher RD, Fisher SG, et al. Amiodarone in patients with congestive heart failure and asymptomatic ventricular arrhythmia. N Engl J Med 1995;333:77-82.

[83] Cairns JA, Connolly SJ, Roberts R, et al. Randomised trial of outcome after myocardial infarction in patients with frequent or repetitive ventricular premature depolarisations: CAMIAT. Lancet 1997;349:675-682.

[84] Herre J, Sauve M, Malone P, et al. Long-term results of amiodarone therapy in patients with recurrent sustained ventricular tachycardia or ventricular fibrillation. J Am Coll Cardiol 1989;13:442-449.

[85] Julian DG, Camm AJ, Frangin G, et al. Randomised trial of effect of amiodarone on mortality in patients with left-ventricular dysfunction after recent myocardial infarction: EMIAT. Lancet 1997;349:667-674.

[86] Bardy GH, Lee KL, Mark DB, et al. Amiodarone or an implantable cardioverter-defibrillator for congestive heart failure. N Engl J Med 2005;352:225-237.

[87] Makikallio TH, Huikuri HV. Association between usage of beta-blocking medication and benefit from implantable cardioverter therapy. Am J Cardiol 2006;98:1245-1247.

[88] Lai HM, Aronow WS, Kruger A, Dersai H, Amin H, Frishman WH, et al. Effect of beta blockers, angiotensin-converting enzyme inhibitors or angiotensin receptor blockers, and statins on mortality in patients with implantable cardioverter-defibrillators. Am J Cardiol 2008; 102:77-78.

[89] Kruger A, Aronow WS, Lai H, Desai H, Singla A, Frishman WH, et al. Prevalence of appropriate cardioverter-defibrillator shocks in 1038 consecutive patients with implantable cardioverter-defibrillators. Am J Therap 2009; 16:323-325.

[90] O'Rourke RA. Role of myocardial revascularization in sudden cardiac death. Circulation 1992;85(suppl I):I-112-I-117.

[91] Bigger JT Jr, for the Coronary Artery Bypass Graft (CABG) Patch Trial Investigators. Prophylactic use of implanted cardiac defibrillators in patients at high risk for ventricular arrhythmias after coronary artery bypass graft surgery. N Engl J Med 1997;337:1569-1575.

[92] Platia EV, Griffith LSC, Watkins L Jr, et al. Treatment of malignant ventricular arrhythmias with endocardial resection and implantation of the automatic cardioverter-defibrillator. N Engl J Med 1986;314:213-216.

[93] Tresch DD, Platia EV, Guarnieri T, et al. Refractory symptomatic ventricular tachycardia and venricular fibrillation in elderly patients. Am J Med 1987;83:399-404.

[94] Tresch DD, Troup PJ, Thakur RK, et al. Comparison of efficacy of automatic implantable cardioverter defibrillator in patients older and younger than 65 years of age. Am J Med 1991;90:717-724.

[95] Rastegar H, Link MS, Foote CB, et al. Perioperative and long-term results with mapping-guided subendocardial resection and left ventricular endoaneurysmorrhaphy. Circulation 1996;94:1041-1048.

[96] Morady F, Harvey M, Kalbfleisch SJ, et al. Radiofrequency catheter ablation of ventricular tachycardia in patients with coronary artery disease. Circulation 1993;87:363-372.

[97] Gonska B-D, Cao K, Schaumann A, et al. Catheter ablation of ventricular tachycardia in 136 patients with coronary artery disease: Results and long-term follow-up. J Am Coll Cardiol 1994;24:1506-1514.

[98] Channamsetty V, Aronow WS, Sorbera C, et al. Efficacy of radiofrequency catheter ablation in treatment of elderly patients with supraventricular tachyarrhythmias and ventricular tachycardia. Am J Therap 2006; 13: 513-515.

http://dx.doi.org/10.5772/57545

[99] Kuck K-H, Schaumann A, Eckardt L, et al. Catheter ablation of stable ventricular tachycardia before defibrillator implantation in patients with coronary heart disease (VTACH): a multicentre randomised controlled trial. Lancet 2010; 375: 31-40.

[100] Moss AJ, Hall WJ, Cannom DS, et al. Improved survival with an implanted defibrillator in patients with coronary disease at high risk for ventricular arrhythmia. N Engl J Med 1996;335:1933-1940.

[101] The Antiarrhythmics versus Implantable Defibrillators (AVID) Investigators. A comparison of antiarrhythmic-drug therapy with implantable defibrillators in patients resuscitated from near-fatal ventricular arrhythmias. N Engl J Med 1997;337:1576-1583.

[102] Roy D, Green M, Talajic M, et al. Mode of death in the Canadian Implantable Defibrillator Study (CIDS) (abstract). Circulation 1998;98(suppl I):1-495.

[103] Bokhari F, Newman D, Greene M, et al. Long-term comparison of the implantable cardioverter defibrillator versus amiodarone. Eleven-year follow-up of a subset of patients in the Canadian Implantable Defibrillator Study CIDS. Circulation 2004;110:112-116.

[104] Siebels J, Cappato R, Ruppel R, et al. Preliminary results of the Cardiac Arrest Study Hamburg (CASH). Am J Cardiol 1993;72:109F-113F.

[105] Cappato R, Siebels J, Kuck KH. Value of programmed electrical stimulation to predict clinical outcome in the Cardiac Arrest Study Hamburg (CASH) (abstract). Circulation 1998;98(suppl I):I-495-I-496.

[106] Buxton AE, Lee KL, Fisher JD, et al. A randomized study of the prevention of sudden death in patients with coronary artery disease. N Engl J Med 1999;341:1882-1890.

[107] Moss AJ, Zareba W, Hall WJ, et al. Prophylactic implantation of a defibrillator in patients with myocardial infarction and reduced ejection fraction. N Engl J Med 2002;346:877-883.

[108] Goldenberg I, Moss AJ. Treatment of arrhythmias and use of implantable cardioverter-defibrillators to improve survival in elderly patients with cardiac disease. In Aronow WS (ed): Clinics in Geriatric Medicine on Heart Failure, Philadelphia, Elsevier, 2007; 23:205-219.

[109] Kaplan BA, Epstein LM, Albert CM, Stevenson WG. Survival in octogenarians receiving implantable defibrillators. Am Heart J 2006;152:714-719.

[110] Goldenberg I, Gillespie J, Moss AJ, et al. Long-term benefit of primary prevention with an implantable cardioverter-defibrillator. An extended 8-year follow-up study of the MulticenterAutomatic Defibrillator Implantation Trial II. Circulation 2010; 122: 1265-1271.

[111] Seidl K, Hauer B, Schwick NG, et al. Comparison of metoprolol and sotalol in preventing ventricular tachyarrhythmias after the implantation of a cardioverter/defibrillator. Am J Cardiol 1998;82:744-748.

[112] Brodine WN, Tung RT, Lee JK, et al. Effects of beta-blockers on implantable cardioverter defibrillator therapy and survival in the patients with ischemic cardiomyopathy (from the Multicenter Automatic Defibrillator Implantation Trial-II. Am J Cardiol 2005;96:691-695.

[113] Epstein AE, DiMarco JP, Ellenbogen KA, Estes NA 3rd, Freedman RA, Gettes LS, et al. ACC/AHA/HRS Guidelines for Device-Based Therapy of Cardiac Rhythm Abnormalities: Executive Summary. A Report of the American College of Cardiology/ American Heart Association Task Force on Practice Guidelines (Writing Committee to Revise the ACC/AHA/NASPE 2002 Guideline Update for Implantation of Cardiac Pacemakers and Antiarrhythmia Devices). Developed in collaboration with the American Association for Thoracic Surgery and Society of Thoracic Surgeons. J Am Coll Cardiol 2008; 51:2085-2105

[114] Jessup M, Abraham WT, Casey DE, et al. 2009 focused update: ACCF/AHA guidelines for the diagnosis and management of heart failure in adults. A Report of the American College of Cardiology Foundation/American Heart Association Task Force on Practice Guidelines. Developed in collaboration with the International Society for Heart and Lung Transplantation. J Am Coll Cardiol 2009; 53: 1343-1382..

[115] Bristow MR, Saxon LA, Boehmer J, et al. Cardiac-resynchronization therapy with or without an implantable defibrillator in advanced chronic heart failure. N Eng J Med 2004; 350: 2140-2150.

[116] Maron BJ, Shen W-K, Link MS, et al. Efficacy of implantable cardioverter-defibrillators for the prevention of sudden death in patients with hypertrophic cardiomyopathy. N Engl J Med 2000;342:365-373.

[117] Brugada P, Brugada R, Brugada J, Geelen P. Use of the prophylactic implantable cardioverter defibrillator for patients with normal hearts. Am J Cardiol 1999;83:98D-100D.

[118] LeLorier P, Krahn AD, Klein GJ, et al. Comparison of patients with syncope with left ventricular dysfunction and negative electrophysiologic testing to cardiac arrest survivors and patients with syncope and preserved left ventricular function and impact of an implantable defibrillator. Am J Cardiol 2002;90:77-79.

[119] Lorga-Filho A,, Geelen P, Vanderheyden M, et al. Early benefit of implantable cardioverter defibrillator therapy in patients waiting for cardiac transplantation. Pacing Clin Electrophysiol 1998;21:1747-1751.

[120] Aronow WS, Sorbera C, Chagarlamudi A, et al. Indications for and long-term survival in patients with automatic implantable cardioverter-defibrillators. Cardiol Rev 2005;13:50-51.

[121] Hohnloser SH, Kuck KH, Dorian P, et al. Prophylactic use of an implantable cardioverter-defibrillator after acute myocardial infarction. N Engl J Med 2004;351:2481-2488.

[122] Steinbeck G, Andresen D, Seidl K, et al. Defibrillator implantation early after myocardial infarction. N Engl J Med 2009; 361: 1427-1436.

[123] Dorian P, Hohnloser SH, Thorpe KE, et al. Mechanisms underlying the lack of effect of implantable cardioverter-defibrillator therapy on mortality in hgh-risk patients with recent myocardial infarction. Insights from the Defibrillation in Acute Myocardial Infarction trial (DINAMIT). Circulation 2010; 122: 2645-2652.

[124] Desai H, Aronow WS, Tsai FS, et al. Statins reduce appropriate cardioverter-defibrillator shocks and mortality in patients with heart failure and combined cardiac resynchronization and implantable cardioverter-defibrillator therapy. J Cardiovasc Pharmacol Therap 2009; 14:176-179.

[125] Desai H, Aronow WS, Ahn C, Tsai FS, et al. Incidence of appropriate cardioverter-defibrillator shocks and mortality in patients with heart failure treated with combined cardiac resynchronization therapy plus implantable cardioverter-defibrillator therapy versus implantable cardioverter-defibrillator therapy. J Cardiovasc Pharmacol Therap 2010; 15:37-40.

[126] Desai H, Aronow WS, Ahn C, Gandhi K, Hussain S, Lai HM, et al. Risk factors for appropriate cardioverter-shocks, inappropriate cardioverter shocks, and time to mortality in 549 patients with heart failure. Am J Cardiol 2010; 105:1336-1338.

[127] Gandhi K, Aronow WS, Desai H, Amin H, Lai HM, Frishman WH, et al. Incidence of appropriate cardioverter-defibrillator shocks and mortality in patients with implantable cardioverter-defibrillators with ischemic cardiomyopathy versus nonischemic cardiomyopathy at 33-month follow-up. Arch Med Sci 2010; 6:900-903.

[128] Tsai F, Aronow WS, Devabhaktuni S, Desai H, Kruger A, Lai HM, et al. Prevalence of complications during implantation and during 38-month follow-up of 1060 consecutive patients with implantable cardioverterr-defibrillators. Am J Therap 2010; 17: e8-e10.

[129] Swerdlow CD, Gunderson BD, Ousdigian KT, Abeyatne A, Stadler RW, Gillberg JM, et al. Downloadable algorithm to reduce inappropriate shocks caused by fractures of implantable cardioverter-defibrillator leads. Circulation 2008; 118: 2122-2129.

[130] Rienstra M, Smit MD, Nieuwland W, et al. Persistent atrial fibrillation is associated with appropriate shocks and heart failure in patients with left ventricular dysfunction treated with an implantable cardioverter defibrillator. Am Heart J 2007; 153: 120-126.

[131] Daubert JP, Zareba W, Cannom DS, et al. Inappropriate implantable cardioverter-defibrillator shocks in MADIT II. Frequency, mechanisms, predictors, and survival impact. J Am Coll Cardiol 2008; 51: 1357-1365.

[132] Santini M, Gasparini M, Landolina M, et al. Device-detected atrial tachyarrhythmias predict adverse outcome in real-world patients with implantable biventricular defibrillators. J Am Coll Cardiol 2011; 57: 167-172.

[133] Hager CS, Jain S, Blackwell J, et al. Effect of renal function on survival after implantable cardioverter defibrillator placement. Am J Cardiol 2010; 106: 1297-1300.

[134] Mainigi SK, Almuti K, Figueredo VM, et al. Usefulness of radiofrequency ablation of supraventricular tachycardia to decrease inappropriate shocks from implantable cardioverter-defibrillators. Am J Cardiol 2012; 109: 231-237

[135] The DAVID Trial Investigators. Dual-chamber pacing or ventricular backup pacing in patients with an implantable defibrillator. The Dual Chamber and VVI Implantable Defibrillator (DAVID) Trial. JAMA 2002;288:3115-3123.

[136] Sukhija R, Aronow WS, Sorbera C, et al. Patients, mean age 70 years, with dual-chamber rate-responsive pacing (DDDR-70) have a higher mortality than patients with backup ventricular pacing (VVI-40) at 3.7-year follow-up. J Gerontol: Med Sci 2005;60A:M603-M604.

[137] Sukhija R, Aronow WS, Sorbera C, et al. Left ventricular ejection fraction and prevalence of new left ventricular wall motion abnormality at long-term follow-up in patients treated with dual-chamber rate-responsive pacing at a rate of 70/minute versus backup ventricular pacing at a rate of 40/minute. Am J Cardiol 2005;96:412-413.

[138] Sukhija R, Aronow WS, Sorbera C, et al. Mortality, left ventricular ejection fraction, and prevalence of new left ventricular wall motion abnormality in patients with implantable cardioverter-defibrillators treated with biventricular pacing versus right venricular pacing. Am J Therap 2007;14:328-330.

[139] Buber J, Goldenberg I, Moss AJ, et al. Reduction in life-threatening ventricular tachyarrhythmias in statin-treated patients with nonischemic cardiomyopathy enrolled in the MADIT-CRT (Multicenter Automatic Defibrillator Implantation Trial with Cardiac Resynchronization Therapy). J Am Coll Cardiol 2012; 60: 749-755.

[140] Ouellet G, Huang DT, Moss AJ, et al. Effect of cardiac resynchronization therapy on the risk of first and recurrent ventricular tachyarrhythmic events in MADIT-CRT. J Am Coll Cardiol 2012; 60: 1809-1816..

[141] Moss AJ, Schuger C, Beck CA, et al. Reduction in inappropriate therapy and mortality through ICD programming. N Engl J Med 2012; 367: 2275-2283.

[142] Gasparini M, Proclemer A, Klersy C, et al. Effect of long-detection interval vs standard-detection interval for implantable cardioverter-defibrillators on antitachycardia

pacing and shock delivery. The ADVANCE III randomized clinical trial. JAMA 2013; 309: 1903-1911.

[143] Yung D, Birnie D, Dorian P, et al. Survival after implantable cardioverter-defibrillator implantation in the elderly. Circulation 2013; 127: 2383-2392.

[144] Al-Khatib SM, Hellkamp A, Bardy GH, et al. Survival of patients receiving a primary prevention implantable cardioverter-defibrillator in clinical practice vs clinical trials. JAMA 2013; 309: 55-62.

[145] Powel BD, Saxon LA, Boehmer JP, et al. Survival after shock therapy in implantable cardioverter-defibrillator and cardiac resynchronization therapy-defibrillator receipients according to rhythm shocked. The ALTITUDE Survival by Rhythm Study. J Am Coll Cardiol 2013; 62: 1674-1679.

Chapter 6

Surgery for Atrial Fibrillation: An Overview

Haralabos Parissis, B.C. Ramesh and Bassel Al-Alao

Additional information is available at the end of the chapter

http://dx.doi.org/10.5772/57421

1. Introduction

Atrial Fibrillation (AF) is the commonest cardiac arrhythmia. The Epidemiology of the disease is presented in Figure 1.

- **Affects 0.4% of general population**
- **2.2 million people in US are in AF**
- **AF accounts for 1/3 of arrhythmia hospitalizations**
- **Predominantly a disease of the elderly**
- **Men more frequently affected than women even after adjustment for all other risk factors**
- **The number of patients with AF is likely to increase 2.5 fold over the next 50 years**

Figure 1. Epidemiology of Atrial Fibrillation

AF is usually associated with underlying cardiovascular disorders, however in around 30% of the cases, AF occurs alone.

Atrial Fibrillation occurs when high rate depolarizing waves conduct through different lesion pathways into the atrium leading to asynchronous contraction of atrial wall segments. This will conduct irregularly through the AV node giving irregular ventricular response rate. This asynchronous contraction prevents effective atrial contraction resulting in residual stagnant blood in the chambers leading to thrombus formation which can break off causing CVA. Furthermore, there is a decrease in cardiac output due to loss of atrial kick, which contribute up to 30% of forward cardiac output especially during periods of diastolic dysfunction.

There is an increasing incidence with age and sex as per Figure 2.

INTECH
open science | open minds

© 2014 Parissis et al.; licensee InTech. This is a paper distributed under the terms of the Creative Commons Attribution License (http://creativecommons.org/licenses/by/3.0), which permits unrestricted use, distribution, and reproduction in any medium, provided the original work is properly cited.

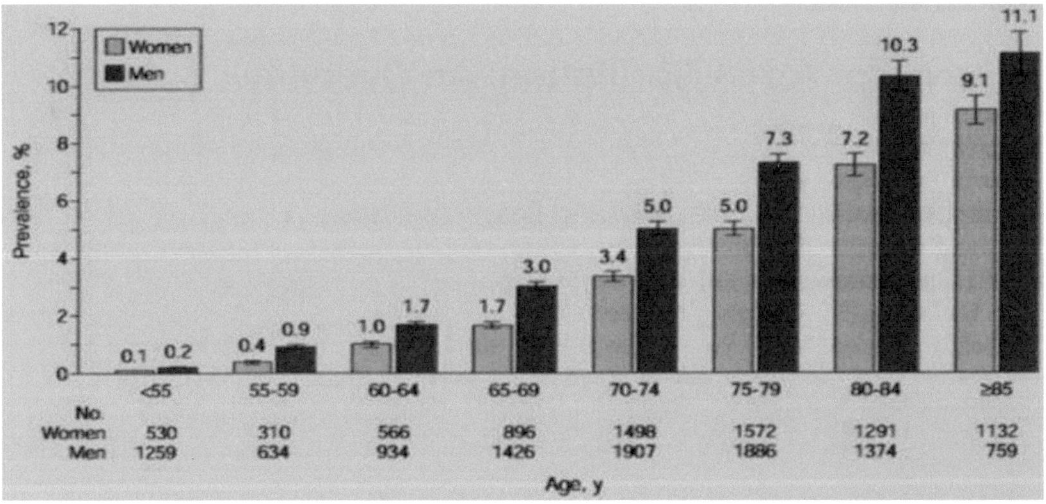

Figure 2. Prevalence of diagnosed atrial fibrillation stratified by age and sex.

Classification of Atrial Fibrillation as per Figure 3:

1. Isolated: A Single episode of AF
2. Recurrent: If more than 2 episodes of AF
3. Paroxysmal: Self-limited bouts of AF
4. Persistent: Requires drugs-DC version
5. Permanent: Non-revertable AF

2. Significance of AF

AF contributes significantly to cardiovascular morbidity and mortality [1].

AF consists off an independent risk factor for death (RR 1.5 – 1.9). There is a link between AF and Thromboembolism [2] :there is a 5 times increased risk of CVA in patients with AF. The presence of rheumatic valvular disease increases the risk of CVA 17-fold. Ultimately AF is responsible for 15% of all CVAs.

Moreover, conventional medical therapy for AF is unsatisfactory because the failure rate is 50% at 1 year and 85% at 2 years. There is a haemorrhagic risk with the use of warfarin for AF and finally antiarrhythmic agents are not specific for atrial activity.

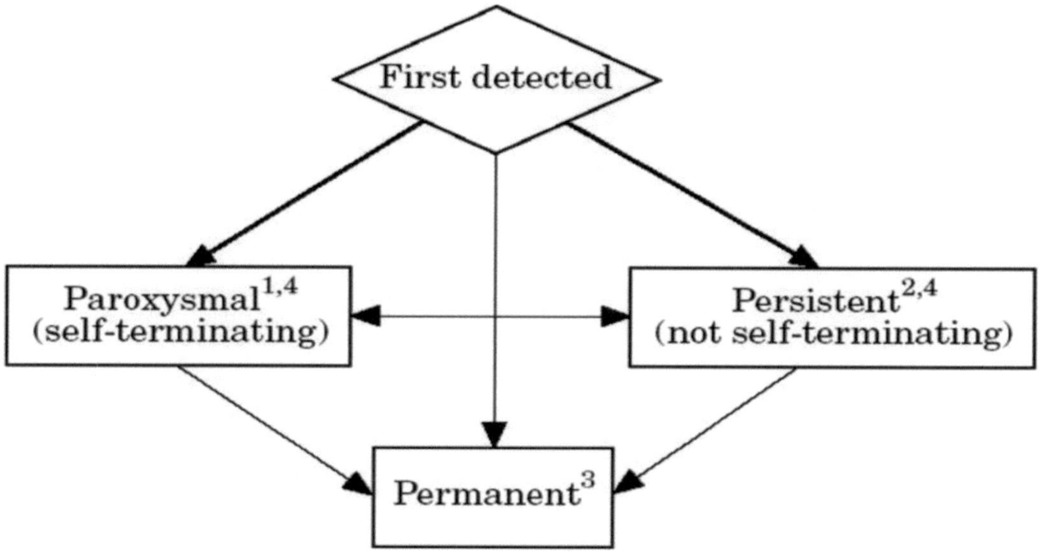

Figure 3. Patterns of atrial fibrillation. (1) episodes that generally last less than or equal to 7 days (most less than 24h; (2) usually more than 7 days; (3) cardioversion faild or not attempted; and (4) either paroxysmal or persistent AF may be recurrent.

3. Pathophysiology of AF

1. Historically in 1962, Moe's developed the "multiple wandering wavelet" hypothesis.
2. Allessie in 1995 eluded on the principles of electrophysiologic changes and electrical remodelling during AF due to:
   a. Intracellular calcium loading.
   b. Down-regulated Ca channel activity.
   c. ↓ Action potential duration.
   d. Shorter refractory period in left atrial tissue.

The functional requirements for re-entrant arrhythmias are: 1) Tissue substrate to support re-entrant excitation, 2) Area of unidirectional block and 3) Typically areas of slow conduction as depicted in Figure 4.

1. It was finally noted that AF begets AF [3].
2. The importance of primary local generator single re-entry circuits was somehow proved with the concept of surgical interruption of macro-re-entrant circuits with the Cox-Maze procedure.
3. Finally, Haissaguerre in 1998 [4] showed that paroxysmal AF originates from ectopic foci in the pulmonary veins.

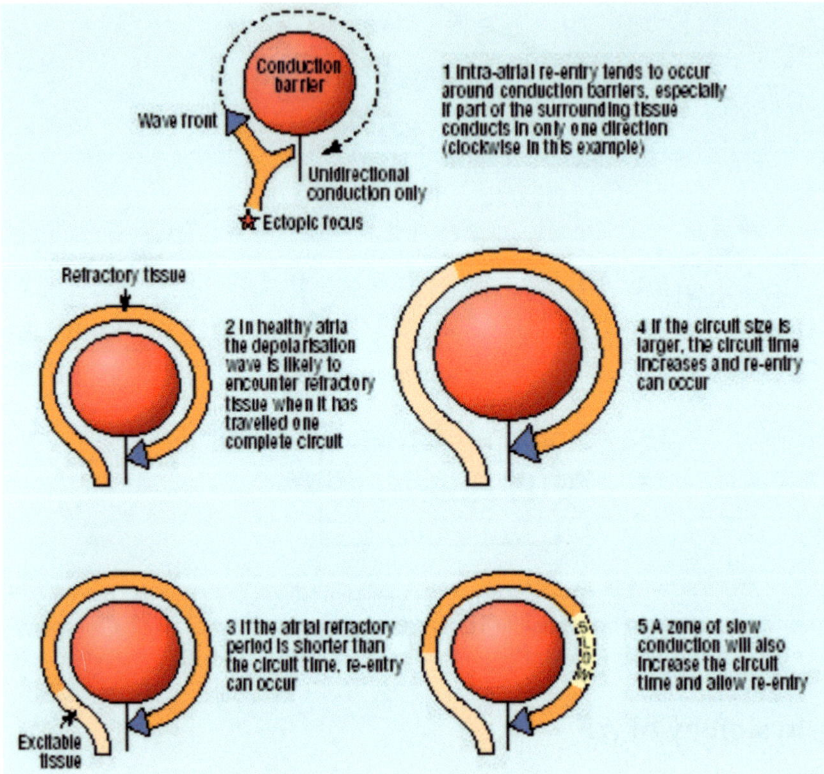

Figure 4. The functional requirements for re-entrant arrhythmias

The minimum diagnostic work-up of an AF patient is presented in Figure 5.

(1) History and physical examination
- 1.1 Define the presence and nature of symptoms
- 1.2 Define the clinical type of atrial fibrillation: paroxysmal, chronic or recent onset
- 1.3 Define the onset of the first symptomatic attack and/or date of discovery of atrial fibrillation.
- 1.4 Define the frequency, duration (shortest and longest episodes), precipitating factors and modes of termination (self-terminating versus persistent) of symptomatic episodes.
- 1.5 Define the presence of an underlying heart disease or other possible identifiable cause (e.g. alcohol consumption, diabetes, hyperthyroidism) which could be cured.

(2) Electrocardiogram
- 2.1 Left ventricular hypertrophy
- 2.2 Duration and morphology of the P waves in sinus rhythm
- 2.3 Evidence of repolarisation changes, bundle branch block, old myocardial infarction and other abnormality.

(3) Echocardiogram (M mode and bidimentional)
- 3.1 Evidence and type of underlying heart disease
- 3.2 Size of the left atrium
- 3.3 Left ventricular size and function
- 3.3 Left ventricular hypertrophy
- 3.4 Intracavitary thrombus (poor sensitivity).

(4) Thyroid test function

If first discovery of atrial fibrillation, if the ventricular rate is difficult to control or if amiodarone has been used in the past.

Figure 5. The minimum diagnostic work-up of an AF patient

http://dx.doi.org/10.5772/57421

4. Surgery for AF

The idea of creating a corridor-link between the sinus node and atrio-ventricular node that could potentially restore regular rhythm became the base of the surgical treatment of AF.

The principles of surgery for AF, takes into account:

- Incisions and creation of lesions in the atria to interrupt macro-re-entrant circuits.
- Creation of blind alleys for atrial electrical activation.
- Appendage excision.

The procedure consists of an open-heart surgical approach, as described by James Cox, namely making linear lesions in the right and left atria to prevent the occurrence of multiple reentering circuits.

Based on mapping studies of animal and human AF, Cox and colleagues [5] developed a surgical procedure (Cox maze procedure) that controls AF in more than 90% of selected patients. In the original procedure atrial appendages are excised and the pulmonary veins are isolated. Appropriately placed atrial incisions not only interrupt the conduction routes of the most common re-entrant circuits, but they also direct the sinus impulse from the surgical ablation node to the atrio-ventricular node along a specified route.

Although encouraging and successful results were obtained, the original surgical technique, the Cox maze I procedure, was modified to become the Cox maze II procedure because of late chrono-tropic problems with the surgical ablation node and intra-atrial conduction delays that resulted in diminished left atrial contraction. However the Cox maze II procedure proved to be technically difficult to perform. As a result, it was modified to become the Cox maze III procedure, which soon became the surgical technique of choice for the treatment of medically resistant AF.

The results of the Cox Maze III (cut and sew) showed that in 346 patients, the operative mortality were less than 2%. The AF was cured in >90-95% of the cases. Left and right atrial function was restored in 93% and 99% of patients correspondingly. 15 % of the patients required pacemakers. Long-term CVA was very low at 0.1% per year [5, 6].

Temporary postoperative AF was frequent, presenting in 38% of patients. This problem was related to a shortened atrial refractory period during the procedure and did not preclude long-term success. Successful ablation treatment of AF was independent of mitral valve disease, type of AF, and left atrial size.

So, although concomitant organic heart disease did not decrease the effectiveness of the Cox maze III procedure in the series of Cox and colleagues, Gillinov et al [7] demonstrated decreased success rate in their study. In most series, concomitant mitral valve surgery with the Cox maze III procedure cured AF in 75% to 82% of patients.

5. Beyond the Cox-Maze III

The Cox-Maze III (cut and sew as seen in Figure 6) perceived complexity, is time-consuming and requires CPB and aortic cross clamp. A systematic review by Khargi et al [8] and a comparative study by Chiappini et al [9] concluded that there was not any significant difference in the postoperative SR conversion rates between the classical 'cut and sew' and the alternative sources of energy, which were used to treat atrial fibrillation.

Therefore, during the last decade AF surgery was popularized with simpler operations, by performing only LA maze (Figure 7) and using alternate energy sources for trans-mural lesions to produce lines of conduction block speedily with minor risk of bleeding.

Of note, during LA ablation one performs pulmonary vein isolation, LA appendage resection, possibly LA appendage to left PV lesion and lastly a PV connecting to MV annulus (mitral) lesion.

Table 1 shows the results of LA maze using different energy sources and Table 2 shows the characteristics and differences between 3 widely used energy sources.

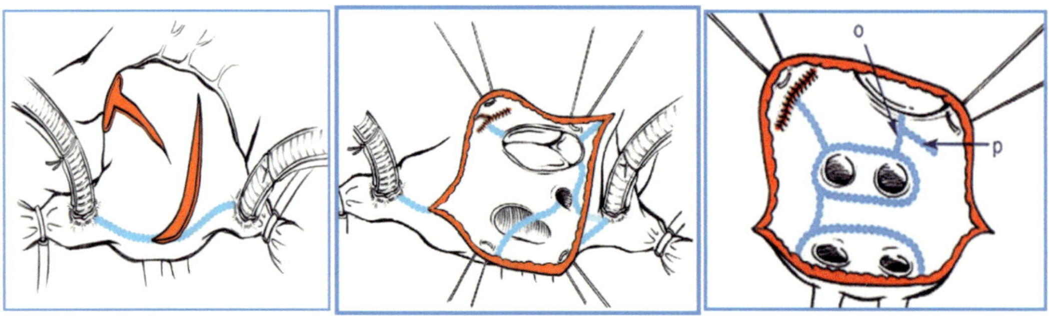

Figure 6. RA and LA Maze (Cox –Maze III)

Author	Year	Number of Patients	Lesion Type	%Sinus Rhythm mid/long-term follow-up
Sie	2004	200	RF	80
Kondo	2003	31	Cryoablation, RF	79.3
Kress	2002	23	RF	86
Wellens	2002	30	RF	65
Guden	2002	23	RF	81
Benussi	2002	132	Epicardial RF	77
Deneke	2002	21	RF	82
Mohr	2002	234	RF	81.1
Knaut	2002	105	Microwave	61
Pasic	2001	48	RF	92

Table 1. Left atrial Maze: Results of contemporary publications, using various energy sources.

http://dx.doi.org/10.5772/57421

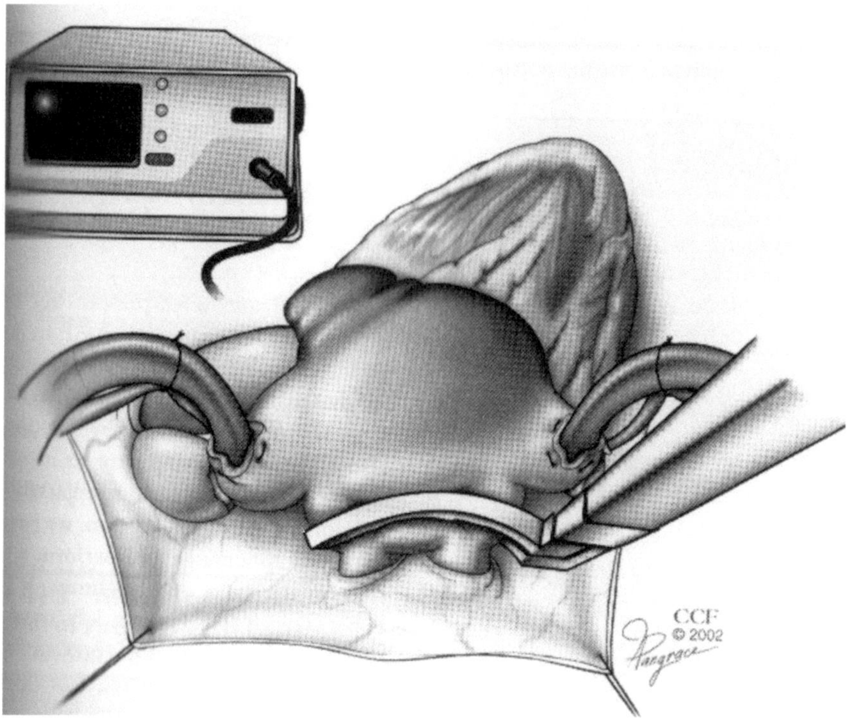

Figure 7. LA maze using alternate energy sources

Radiofrequency	Microwave	Cryothermy
Current of 350 kHz – 1 MHz. Hyperthermic lesions cause a loss of cellular excitability at 50°C.	High frequency electromagnetic radiation causes oscillation of water molecules.	The mechanism of cryogenic tissue injury in the early phase is actually organelle and mitochondrial dysfunction and subsequent edema and cell necrosis upon thawing.
The temperature must remain below 100°C to prevent cavitation.	The oscillation of the water produces kinetic energy and subsequent heat, a process called dielectric heating. The AFx Microwave device can produce an endocardial ablation by reaching a goal temperature of 50° at 5 mm after 25 seconds. The same device produces an epicardial ablation at 45 seconds using a slightly higher wattage	With the early Frigitronics nitrous oxide based systems, a temperature of −55°C had to be maintained for two minutes, and repeated exposures were sometimes required. Newer, argon-based systems provide cooler temperatures that may permit effective ablations in 45 seconds or less.
Radiofrequency energy ablation is very similar to standard electro-cautery. Although there are bipolar and irrigated unipolar RF options, RF is generally unipolar and uses very fast AC current, which avoids depolarizing the heart. The mechanism is resistive of ohmic heating, which involves the concentration of a large amount of energy on a small surface area. The energy disperses to the ground pad, but the area where it is focused is heated, resulting in ablation. It is		

Radiofrequency	Microwave	Cryothermy
possible to control both temperature and energy. Energy control will permit precise application of, say, 50 watts, but temperature is not controlled. Temperature control allows the device to maintain a precise goal temperature.		
Lesion depths 3-6 mm	Increased depth and volume of heated tissue	Nirous oxide based cryoprobe
Unipolar or Bipolar •bipolar concentrates energy between electrodes –easy, quick, narrow lesions •irrigation delays micro bubble formation –accurate lesion monitoring •maximally flexible –handle designed for access and visibility –malleable electrodes for any heart size/shape –jaw head pitch and roll adaptive transmurality	Less charring, but less flexible compare with Radiofrequency.	Difficulty with inflexibility of probes
Unipolar: unfocused energy delivery	Risk of damage to surrounding tissues	There is no tissue vaporization or charring
Surface charring may cause thromboembolic complications		The endocardial surface remains smooth
Saline cooled systems improve charring		
Heat is conducted to surrounding tissues (risk of damage, e.g. oesophageal perforation)		
"How do I know I am done"? 1) Heating of cells creates a shift in intracellular fluid to extra-cellular space 2) Creates a drop in impedance 3) Algorithm monitors changes in impedance		

Table 2. Various energy sources/ Characteristics and properties

6. Recent important advances in AF surgery

The mid- and long-term success rate is in the 80% range. This has prompted various authorities to popularized adding Maze procedures to concomitant cardiac surgery; with the view to potentially treat AF with a simple, short and less invasive procedure. Moreover, minimal access pulmonary vein isolation has been currently implemented for "lone" AFib or as part of a mini-Mitral approach.

Wolf et al [10, 11], reported on 27 patients (22Males, mean age 57) who underwent Bilateral thoracoscopic PVI and LAA excision for AFib (18 paroxysmal, 4 persistent, 5 permanent AFib). There were no conversions or major complications. There was 91% freedom from AF at 3 months follow-up. The authors concluded that bilateral video-assisted thoracoscopic pulmonary vein isolation with excision of the left atrial appendage is feasible and safe and offers a promising, new, minimally invasive, beating-heart approach for curative surgical treatment of atrial fibrillation.

Jeanmart et al [12] evaluate their practice with the association of the mini-maze procedure, done with the use of the Cardioblade pen, and concomitant minimally invasive mitral valve surgery. They studied 103 patients. 41% had intermittent and 59% permanent AFib. At mean follow up of 17 months, 70% of the patients studied were in Sinus Rhythm and 2% were pacemaker dependent. The authors concluded that the use of unipolar radiofrequency ablation to perform a mini-maze during minimally invasive mitral valve surgery is a safe procedure and is associated with good early results.

7. Postoperative AFib

Post-operative AFib is different to conventional AF (micro- versus macro-re-entrant circuits). Moreover the local refractory periods may be shorter and re-entrant circuits can be smaller. Post-operative AFib is common after open-heart surgery (30-50%) and it must be treated with anti-arrhythmics and anticoagulation, if it persists more than 48 hours. Warfarin should be continued on all patients for at least 3 months and lastly in patients who remain in AFib for 6 weeks, cardio-version is essential.

If AF with concomitant cardiac surgery	"Lone" AF (for younger patients with limiting symptoms, Contraindication to anticoagulation, Thromboembolic stroke while on anti-coagulation)
Paroxysmal or persistent AF: PVI and LAA excision	Paroxysmal or persistent AF: minimally invasive PVI and LAA excision
Permanent AF: left Maze (PVI, LA connecting lesions and LAA excision) and Right side Maze	Permanent AF: left Maze or Cox-Maze III

Table 3. Strategies for the surgical treatment of AF

8. Conclusions

Regardless of the method used, the goals remain the same. The lesions should, ideally, be transmural; when minimally invasive procedures are implemented, the lesions should proceed from the epicardium of the beating heart, which changes the physics of many of the lesions. The method must also allow for tissues of variable thickness and characteristics, as a patient with rheumatic atrial pathology will have a much more difficult atrium to ablate than a coronary bypass patient.

A natural question arises as to which lesion pattern surgeons should be using. There probably isn't a simple answer to this question, because:

a. Data on lesion set efficacy is influenced by patient variables such as left atrial diameter, duration of preoperative atrial fibrillation, coexisting pathology etc.

b. Comparing the efficacy of one lesion pattern to another in clinical trials will require too many patients in each treatment arm to achieve statistical power.

c. Not all lesion patterns can be effectively or safely delivered with all energy sources.

Table 3, represents our policy of implementing strategies for the surgical treatment of AF. By enlarge; the right atrium has a longer effective refractory period than the left atrium and in general sustains only longer reentry circuits, the most common being the counterclockwise circuit of typical atrial flutter. Atrial flutter can be ablated, by a trans-mural lesion connecting the tricuspid annulus to the IVC; additional lesions connecting a lateral right atriotomy to the IVC or coronary sinus to the IVC is occasionally necessary to ablate an atypical right atrial flutter.

In summary, in patients with persistent or permanent AF who present for cardiac surgery, the addition of surgical AF ablation led to a significantly higher rate of sinus rhythm in RCT and non-RCT studies compared with cardiac surgery alone, and this effect remains robust over the longer term (1-5 years). Although non-RCT studies suggest the possibility of reduced risk of stroke and death, this remains to be proven in prospective RCTs with adequate power and follow-up [13, 14].

9. The future

Further refinements in energy sources, lesion sets, minimally invasive techniques will be developed. Routine preoperative EP screening and better understanding of selection criteria will improve success rates. That may be achieved with close collaboration with EP cardiologists.

The up till now results are encouraging therefore minimally invasive PVI may be routinely considered in all cardiac surgical departments. Lastly, Left atrial maze should become standard treatment of persistent/permanent "lone" AF in selected patients, especially where EP techniques fail.

http://dx.doi.org/10.5772/57421

Author details

Haralabos Parissis[1], B.C. Ramesh[2] and Bassel Al-Alao[1]

1 Cardiothoracic Department, Royal Victoria Hospital, Belfast, UK

2 Cardiopulmonary Transplantation Department, Freeman Hospital, Newcastle Upon Tyne, UK

References

[1] Mahmood SS, Levy D, Vasan RS, Wang TJ. The Framingham Heart Study and the epidemiology of cardiovascular disease: a historical perspective. Lancet. 2013 Sep 27. PubMed PMID: 24084292.

[2] Lubitz SA, Moser C, Sullivan L, Rienstra M, Fontes JD, Villalon ML, et al. Atrial fibrillation patterns and risks of subsequent stroke, heart failure, or death in the community. Journal of the American Heart Association. 2013 Oct;2(5):e000126. PubMed PMID: 24002369.

[3] Wijffels MC, Kirchhof CJ, Dorland R, Allessie MA. Atrial fibrillation begets atrial fibrillation. A study in awake chronically instrumented goats. Circulation. 1995 Oct 1;92(7):1954-68. PubMed PMID: 7671380.

[4] Haissaguerre M, Jais P, Shah DC, Takahashi A, Hocini M, Quiniou G, et al. Spontaneous initiation of atrial fibrillation by ectopic beats originating in the pulmonary veins. The New England journal of medicine. 1998 Sep 3;339(10):659-66. PubMed PMID: 9725923.

[5] Cox JL, Ad N, Palazzo T, Fitzpatrick S, Suyderhoud JP, DeGroot KW, et al. Current status of the Maze procedure for the treatment of atrial fibrillation. Seminars in thoracic and cardiovascular surgery. 2000 Jan;12(1):15-9. PubMed PMID: 10746917.

[6] Cox JL. Cardiac surgery for arrhythmias. Journal of cardiovascular electrophysiology. 2004 Feb;15(2):250-62. PubMed PMID: 15028063.

[7] Gillinov AM, Blackstone EH, McCarthy PM. Atrial fibrillation: current surgical options and their assessment. The Annals of thoracic surgery. 2002 Dec;74(6):2210-7. PubMed PMID: 12643434.

[8] Khargi K, Hutten BA, Lemke B, Deneke T. Surgical treatment of atrial fibrillation; a systematic review. European journal of cardio-thoracic surgery : official journal of the European Association for Cardio-thoracic Surgery. 2005 Feb;27(2):258-65. PubMed PMID: 15691679.

[9] Chiappini B, Martin-Suarez S, LoForte A, Arpesella G, Di Bartolomeo R, Marinelli G. Cox/Maze III operation versus radiofrequency ablation for the surgical treatment of

atrial fibrillation: a comparative study. The Annals of thoracic surgery. 2004 Jan; 77(1):87-92. PubMed PMID: 14726041.

[10] Wolf RK. Minimally invasive surgical treatment of atrial fibrillation. Seminars in thoracic and cardiovascular surgery. 2007 Winter;19(4):311-8. PubMed PMID: 18395630.

[11] Wolf RK, Schneeberger EW, Osterday R, Miller D, Merrill W, Flege JB, Jr., et al. Video-assisted bilateral pulmonary vein isolation and left atrial appendage exclusion for atrial fibrillation. The Journal of thoracic and cardiovascular surgery. 2005 Sep;130(3): 797-802. PubMed PMID: 16153931.

[12] Jeanmart H, Casselman F, Beelen R, Wellens F, Bakir I, Van Praet F, et al. Modified maze during endoscopic mitral valve surgery: the OLV Clinic experience. The Annals of thoracic surgery. 2006 Nov;82(5):1765-9. PubMed PMID: 17062244.

[13] Bakir I, Casselman FP, Brugada P, Geelen P, Wellens F, Degrieck I, et al. Current strategies in the surgical treatment of atrial fibrillation: review of the literature and Onze Lieve Vrouw Clinic's strategy. The Annals of thoracic surgery. 2007 Jan;83(1): 331-40. PubMed PMID: 17184704.

[14] Cheng DC, Ad N, Martin J, Berglin EE, Chang BC, Doukas G, et al. Surgical ablation for atrial fibrillation in cardiac surgery: a meta-analysis and systematic review. Innovations. 2010 Mar;5(2):84-96. PubMed PMID: 22437354.